I0126679

THE MOONTIME HARMONY WORKBOOK

*A Path to Creating a
Sacred and Harmonious
Menstrual Moontime Cycle*

Donna Wolper

The Moontime Harmony Workbook

© 2015 Donna Wolper

ISBN: 978-1-61170-209-5
Library of Congress Control Number: 2015944778

All rights reserved. No part of this publication may be reproduced, stored in a retrieval system or transmitted in any form or by any means, electronic, mechanical, photocopies, recording or otherwise, without the prior written consent of the author.

Cover art by Gina Giommi.

Printed in the USA and UK on acid-free paper.

Robertson Publishing™
www.RobertsonPublishing.com

To purchase additional copies of this book go to:
amazon.com
barnesandnoble.com

To my children, Avra and Jonah, who have been a constant source of inspiration and love to me their entire lives, whom I cherish deeply in my heart and soul.

And to every Wombyn* who is living on our Mother Earth at this time. May we all return to the source of our Feminine power, a root of which can be accessed through the flow of a harmonious moontime. May we all be blessed and illuminated by the lunar light of the Goddess that dwells within. May we remember how to return to our Divine and Sacred selves, especially during one's moontime flow.

iv

CONTENTS

FOREWORD

I spent many years living in a coastal, jungle, fishing village in Mexico. In those early days, the village did not have any electricity, cars or roads. Even today the village still exists without cars and roads, while the main access is by boat.

I lived there for many years, sometimes with my children, sometimes without. Usually I stayed at least 6 months and each time I began to attune to the harmonies and rhythms of the moon, tides and the natural world. It was through this attunement that my menstrual cycle-my moontime- aligned with the phases of the moon and the information for this book surfaced.

Each year that I returned, more clarity emerged and the rhythms of the *blood mysteries* deepened. I finally became aware of my phases and cycles and their interconnectedness with the moon and nature. I embraced this physical part of myself, while opening up to the Divine within. I became familiar with the signposts that helped me navigate my way into the inner garden of the Goddess and began listening to Her messages. I recognized patterns that could be healed, alignments with the phases of the moon, rhythms that could be charted and followed. Each month I began to come home to myself and realized that if I could, any wombyn could. It became clear that once a wombyn knew and understood how to take these conscious steps, she could connect with this Goddess given gift.

I began to keep track of my physical and emotional changes each month. Once in my moontime, I could let go and travel into my inner world where the veil lifted and the Sacred was revealed. I observed that if I honored that flow, I emerged renewed, felt whole and moved out into the world with more joy, ease and energy. Thus the idea for a *workbook*—a format to keep track, observe, monitor and follow my needs and rhythmic changes—was born.

This is the process that I want to share with every *wombyn** in the hope that I can offer a way to understand and demystify your own moontime cycle. It is by illuminating the knowledge of the patterns of your rhythms, that you can embrace your moontime with the awareness that the Goddess intended.

You'll notice I prefer the spelling of *wombyn** instead of *woman* and use the spelling *wembyn** to denote the plural. I believe that the source of our feminine harmony is connected to our wombs; this spelling helps me to remember that connection.

So may the truth of the *blood mysteries* be alive within every *wombyn* and may this balance ripple out into the entire world!

Donna Wolper
Santa Cruz, CA
May 30, 2015

x

INTRODUCTION

*T*he Moontime Harmony Workbook was created to be used as a *work* or *guide* book to encourage a spiritual wellness during your menstrual cycle. It offers *ideas, suggestions* and moontime related *focuses.* It is **not** meant to be a source of information, but a **source of direction** and **inspiration-**things to think about or do**.**

It is intended to help a wombyn achieve a love and a deeper understanding of her menstrual cycle or moontime. The intention is to illuminate the blessings of the *Blood Mysteries*, the essence of which has been existing in the dark. The goal is to encourage a wombyn to look forward to her monthly cycle because she will know how to be prepared. A wombyn can learn to listen to the voices of her body, emotions and spirit. This will then help her to build the confidence that she needs to know how to trust her own intuitive intelligence and wisdom. This will help to de-mystify and empower her experience.

It is a menstrual map that will aid a wombyn who is lost in painful or undesired moontimes to re-orient her feminine compass so that she can find healing, nurturing and growth each month. It is designed to guide a wombyn for thirteen months, the number of lunar months in a solar year.

Each month has a calendar that you can use to chart and follow your rhythms and needs. Each month has a page or two with spaces to journal, answer questions and places to keep track of your physical and emotional needs. These pages offer guidance to a wombyn to help her achieve balance and awareness of her moontime. It points directions and offers reminders so she can follow her moontime experience. It gives her a place to monitor her moontime needs.

There are suggestions and ideas intended to bring to light a process that will help a wombyn get in touch. It provides spaces to follow your cycles, so you can keep track of what surfaces. This might include keeping an account of what might need to be released or transformed, old negative painful patterns, fears, taboos, or shame. Sources of possible disharmony and pain, once identified, can often be replaced with positive patterns that will unfold a harmonious moontime.

Each month has a focus that reflects a different aspect of the moontime or feminine wellbeing. These focuses are meant to suggest ideas to think about; they are often aspects of the moontime that create disharmony. Negative thoughts, practices or conditionings; often the origin of unwanted or uncomfortable moontimes; are looked at from new, healthy perspectives. It is by creating new inner constructs and releasing old, buried fears, images, or beliefs that you can enter into a lighter, joyful and loving relationship with your period or moontime. Once these old patterns are recognized, they can be healed by being replaced by new, positive patterns that will help to unfold a harmonious moontime.

When the lunar light and phases guide a wombyn's experience, moontimes become a spiritual unfolding and an attunement to the Sacred within. Sacred inner worlds emerge, reflecting, like the light of the moon, your own inner Divine energy or connection with the Goddess. As you align with the Blood Mysteries, the essence of the feminine moontime, intuition becomes stronger. Knowing and trusting yourself and your needs becomes clearer. The knowledge of what you require for healing appears and creativity can soar. A wombyn has this opportunity and gift of connection every month. When you do, it's like coming home to yourself.

It is up to a wombyn to reclaim her wisdom and honor her moontime. We are the ones who have to understand that we deserve quiet time or a private space when our blood flows. In cultures that honored the moon lodge and red tent, not just the wombyn, but the entire community accepted and supported that need.

Our fast paced, modern world has forgotten the importance of allowing a wombyn, in her moontime, to commune and reflect with herself. Happily, I see that there is a growing movement to create red tents all around the world where a wombyn can go in order to peacefully and consciously flow during her moontime. It is an important need and right for the health of every wombyn to be able to freely enter a *moonlodge* each month, because it provides the protection she needs physically and psychically while her blood flows. What benefits a wombyn's life will benefit everyone.

So it is time for both wembyn and men to understand that it is vital to a wombyn's health and wellbeing to be allowed the time and space to pay attention to and listen, with respect, to the needs of her body and emotions each month. It enhances her productivity when a wombyn is allowed to dream, rest, and heal without guilt or stress. A wombyn allowed to commune with the Divine is a stronger and healthier being, more vibrant and alive, and has more energy to give to her family and community, not just herself.

The voice of the feminine must be heard. Not just the feminine that deserves equal pay as men, or equal standards in the military or work force, but the Feminine that creates life. Wembyn need to learn and remember that they are sacred and that the flow of their menstrual blood is sacred, holy and healing. Menstruation is *not* a disease, curse or a syndrome. A syndrome is a collection of symptoms that characterize a disease or abnormality and menstruation is not a disease. It is a natural and healthy part of being a wombyn and the rhythm of procreation.

Moontime is a regular, normal, cyclic occurrence of the female body for the purpose of shedding the old, connecting within, focusing on healing, listening to your spirit, renewing as well as being part of the rhythm of procreation. When these natural rhythms and flows are blocked, it creates disturbances or *syndromes* of pain like PMS.

A wombyn can unblock and remove the sources of those disturbances and give healthy attention to the needs of her body, mind and spirit. Learning and remembering how important it is to provide yourself with proper nutrition, rest and exercise-not just during your moontime-but especially during your moontime, are among some of the tools that will help to unblock what stops or blocks the flow.

It is time to transform the disharmonious pain, shame or guilt into the harmonious, sacred, joyous, and illuminated. It is time to love coming home to your own spirit each month. It is time to accept that drifting and dreaming are part of the rhythm and that it will bring you closer to your unconscious, to the void where the Goddess and Divine dwell within. It is time that we honor and rejoice in our inner connection, which is a source of healing and a path to becoming whole. It is time to remember what the Blood Mysteries are really about. It is time to reclaim the essence of the Moontime and Divine Feminine because this is your birthright!

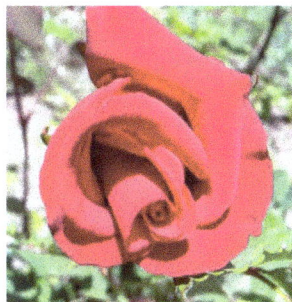

How to Use This Book
and Calendar

This book is intended to be a workbook. It has been created to guide a wombyn for 13 months through different moontime avenues for the purpose of achieving a harmonious moontime.

The workbook comes with thirteen calendars, one for each month in a lunar year. Each solar year has thirteen lunar months, each lunar month has twenty eight days. This occurs because the moon takes twenty eight days to wax and wane from one full moon to the next. Menstrual cycles are often twenty eight-day cycles, in harmony with the waxing and waning of the moon. Each month a wombyn waxes and wanes with physical and emotional rhythms in harmony with the moon.

Each calendar is surrounded by a snake. The snake is a symbol of the Goddess energy. A snake sheds its old skin to make room for its new skin. Each month you shed your blood, you not only shed the lining of your uterus, but you also have the opportunity to shed the old and unused parts of yourself and your life to make way for the new. You also have a psychic door that opens to your Goddess space within where you can journey to revisit your Divine inner world. This is what the symbol of the snake represents.

HOW IS THE CALENDAR MEANT TO BE USED?

On the top of the calendar is a place to put the month and the year. Each month has twenty eight days. Each day is divided into twelve boxes for order and convenience. The first two boxes are meant for the number of the day of that month and the lunar phase that that day is in. The remaining ten boxes can be filled in with personal codes for the things you want to follow. They are used to help you keep track and chart your rhythms and "needs of choice" for every day of the month, not just during your moontime.

There is a chart to write down your personal system of coding so you can keep track of the things that you want to follow each month. The situations that you follow can change month to month or stay the same.

You create the code that you want to use for the need that you want to follow. Some choices are to use color, a code letter or a symbol in that will correspond to a particular need. You can also do a combination or come up with your own language of coding that makes sense to you.

For example, cramps. One of the ten boxes can be used to chart your rhythm of cramps by putting a C or the color navy blue in a box each day that you experience cramping. Many woman have a pattern of cramping and sometimes this pattern can be tracked and even predicted ahead of time. Is that pattern random or predictable? Can you alleviate it if you know ahead of time and perhaps be prepared to take an herb or vitamin that might help? Maybe it is an alert to change your diet a few days before your moontime because you've discovered that certain food choices help minimize or eliminate cramps.

Or, maybe you want to chart depression. The letter D can be put in a box or the color gray, an unhappy face, etc. By the end of a few months, once you have visual patterns to look at, it will be possible to observe your own rhythms, follow your ebbs and tides, your waxes and wanes. It will be easier to *see* and monitor the changes that happen in your body, emotions and/or spirit over the course of a month, several months, a year or even the seasons. Hopefully, by observing your predictable patterns and the things you need to pay attention to, you will begin to know what needs nurturing or preparation and when each month that might be. By recognizing what you need to do for yourself to find balance and healing you will be prepared. By being prepared, you will find balance and harmony.

Also included are *thirteen* areas with nine questions and suggestions of things to think about each month. This includes: spaces to journal, a place to write down your dreams, a place for reminders for your needs or path of healing and space to let your creative artistry wander. These questions and spaces are meant to help you keep track of your emotional tides, physical rhythms, patterns, and discoveries. It is a place for keeping track of *moontime* ideas, needs, questions and observations, with spaces to record your personal experiences. These questions are designed to help you get in touch with your unconscious and inner world. The spaces are to be used to record and keep track of the things that you need in order to tend to your physical needs. By tending the garden of your physical needs, you can experience less discomfort. By becoming aware of your psychic life, you can tune into your inner journey. When you *see* or know your *self*, you begin to understand what you may need to include, release, change, create, transform, heal, or just be with each month so that your flow can flow. These situations don't have to be surprises, but can be followed with clarity.

It is by paying attention to your patterns and rhythms throughout the month, the seasons and the year, that you become aware of your personal changes and needs. This awareness will ultimately guide you to be on top of what you have to do to create your personal harmony before and during your moontime flow. When you recognize what is required for you to do for yourself to find balance and healing, you will be prepared. By being prepared, you will create balance and harmony.

For example, maybe winter finds you experiencing more sadness or depression at predictable times of the month, maybe summer releases more sexual energy. Follow your changes, follow your rhythms, mark it all in your calendar and write about it in your workbook. Is there anything you can do or prepare for? Are there any predictable changes you can look forward to or things you will want to avoid? This is where you can chart and follow your personal needs.

The remaining pages are divided into short focuses. Each focus addresses a different aspect of life that might challenge, be helpful to, or influence a wombyn's moontime. Each focus offers thoughts and questions concerning these ideas. There are spaces to fill in your reactions during and at the end of that focus. The purpose of these focuses is to help you to get in touch with your personal, inner world so you will become more aware of your physical and psychic life in order to create more clarity. Creating more clarity creates more harmony.

A focus might offer ideas to remove sources of pain or blockages or it might offer ideas to enhance the moontime experience. Even if your moontime is not one of pain on any level, these tools will help you identify your rhythms so you can further illuminate your moontime awareness and your sacred self.

Once you have a format or structure with which to look within, your moontime can be transformed into an experience of comfort, healing and attunement. Your inner home will be comfortably arranged to meet your needs. Instead of there being an unwanted guest each month, you will be the gracious host that invites her home!

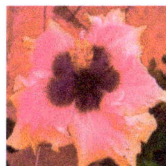

SOME IDEAS for THINGS to CHART and CODE

Bloating	Depression	Days in One's Moontime
Cramps	Food Craving	Irritability, Tensions
Acne	Dreaminess	Breast Tenderness, Changes
Creativity	Headaches	Changing Sleep Patterns
Ovulation	Sexual Changes	Moving In, Out of Moontime
Emotional Changes	Vaginal Changes	Desire to be Alone

Some possibilities for coding your personal needs might be:

Sleep Patterns-S, Cramps-C, Depression-D

Sexual Changes- the color scarlet, Breast Tenderness- the color violet,

Tensions- the color brown

Days in One's Moontime- a red or blue lunar phase, Creativity- a rainbow or paint brush,

Food Craving- an ice cream cone, Dreaminess-clouds.

The choices and codes are yours to create, the needs are yours to follow.

Keep track of your own personal moontime codes here, write them down and know you can change or add to them anytime you need too.

Record your personal moontime codes in the following space.

Symbol or Code	What This Symbol or Code Represents
1.	
2.	
3.	
4.	
5.	
6.	
7.	
8.	
9.	
10.	
11.	
12.	
13.	

Here is an example of what one coded day might look like.

Here is an example of what one week might look like.

IDEAS and SUGGESTIONS
to FOLLOW

*A*t the end of each focus, there are nine places where you can write your personal responses and ideas. The goal is to bring your inner world into the outer world so you can keep track of what is happening to your mind, body, emotions and spirit.

1. Journal - uncensored thoughts, feelings, reactions to this month's moontime.

_____

_____

_____

_____

2. Dreams and Visions - messages from the unconscious, from your Goddess self.

_____

_____

_____

_____

3. Special self-nurturing reminders - things to do for yourself during your moontime, or during the month, to sustain healing.

_____

_____

_____

_____

4. Preparations needed to create a harmonious moontime - reminders for child care, appointments to make or cancel, items to purchase, candles to have for a bath.

_____

_____

_____

_____

5. Reminders for food and diet - when to change or eliminate certain foods, take supplements, herbs to have on hand, things to do that release stress.

_____

_____

_____

_____

6. What old beliefs have been uncovered, need to be eliminated or changed? Create affirmations for transformation.

_____

_____

_____

_____

7. Reminders of activities that will create a harmonious moontime - make an appointment for a massage, walk in nature, get extra sleep, listen to music that you love.

_____

_____

_____

_____

8. What did your last moontime reveal that will help make the next one more spiritual or bring you closer to your sacred self?

_____

_____

_____

_____

9. Create your own ritual, draw or paint your feelings or dreams.

_____

_____

_____

_____

FOCUS #1

LET'S GET STARTED

To Honor One's Moontime Creates and Manifests Order, Balance and Harmony in One's Life

1st month-Menarche

What was your first moontime, your menarche, like? The spirit in which you entered your first moontime often has the power to set a tone for attitudes and expectations of your moontime experience. Negative expectations can create negative experiences. Positive expectations transform into positive experiences. Did your mother or a close female friend or relative explain to you what this 'change' was about? Did she explain what this monthly transformation would be like, explain your newly emerging sexuality. Did she tell you that you could nurture, heal and create life while being a vehicle for Divine energy? Did you know that now you had, as they say in India, "born the flower?"

How did you enter your first moontime or menarche? Were you surrounded by loving wembyn, given gifts, shown how to create rituals to honor your special time of the month? Was there someone who taught you about the rhythm of going within and withdrawing from the outer world in order to let yourself dream and be receptive to visions? And did she explain that these visions might bring answers, suggest solutions or open you to new directions in life?

Hopefully someone was there to tell you how important it is to remember to respect your moontime, your needs, both your inner and outer flows. Might there have been a wise elder who reminded you that squatting on Mother Earth and letting your blood flow onto her was sacred and empowering to you both? That to be in harmony with your moontime teaches you to be in harmony with the cycles of nature, the moon and Mother Earth?

Was your menarche a joyous celebration and a positive affirmation of your entrance into wombyn-hood? Did anyone explain that now you had the power to create life and experience monthly visits to the Goddess' garden of light and dark? Did anyone explain to you that the moon was your sister and that you follow her phases and changes?

Or was your entrance into wombyn-hood unpleasant? Did you look forward to starting your period and yet once she appeared you were confused or disappointed? Was it painful to be *on the rag* and were you embarrassed that now you had the *curse* every month? Did someone say that now *aunt flo* was in town and make you feel like it was a taboo. Were you warned that now you could get pregnant? Did your mother give you a ritualistic slap? How did it feel, smell and make you think or affect your body? Were you ashamed, abandoned, unsupported and uninformed?

In our North American culture, all too often, a girl's first moontime is not honored or celebrated. Most wembyn are left on their own, not mentored by any older, wiser wembyn; given just enough information so they can 'deal' with this new change. If your menarche wasn't sacred and special it may have created a mindset that unfolded into a less than desired moontime.

The good news is that you can replace the original old, painful experiences with positive, joyous affirmations that will tell your unconscious that healing has begun. This healing will filter down to your conscious, corporal body and emotions so that your moontime can become a happily anticipated time of the month.

If you don't know where to begin, here are some questions that might get you started.
1. How did you feel when you entered your menarche? How would you have liked to feel?

2. How supportive were your mother, father, family and friends? How supportive would you have wanted them?

3. Were you confused? In pain? Emotional? What could have made that better?

4. How did you feel about becoming a wombyn? How would you really have wanted to feel?

5. What would the perfect menarche have looked like for you? What didn't happen?

If your menarche was less than perfect and you feel that you may have received some negative programming that has translated into pain or discomfort, you can use the technique of visualization to help reprogram your mind with positive thoughts and feelings.

Find a quiet place and time where you feel comfortable, warm and safe. Relax your whole body using a technique that works for you. Maybe you want to do this the next time you are in your moontime.

When you feel relaxed, using your mind's eye, wander and scan your entire body until you find your womb. Try to imagine what it looks like, feels like, how it smells, what kind of texture it has and what color it is.

Visualize it in your mind's eye. Then look closely and see if there are any dark spots. Look for any places of weakness or illness. If you find any dark or weak areas, ask them why they are there and where they came from. Ask them what you have to do to heal them. Listen to their answers which are often subtle or intuitive. When you have those answers, thank them. Imagine the dark spots, weak areas, imbalances leaving, lightening up and going away. Pay attention to the feelings and thoughts that may surface as the dark transforms into light. Send love to the darkness, send healing and strength to the weakness. Trust yourself.

If it's your emotional world that suffers, look inside your heart and see what confusion it harbors about your moontime. What sorrows might have gotten lodged there? Where did they came from? Offer forgiveness and see them leaving.

Then let your mind wander and visualize the menarche celebration you would have wanted. Who would you have liked to be there? What ceremony or ritual might you have embraced? What wise wisdom would you have liked to have received? From whom? Let your mind and imagination roam freely and see the perfect menarche you would have liked to have, one that is free of shame, guilt or confusion.

Now visualize your womb well, strong, vibrating with life. This is your source of strength and power so see it filled with healing feminine energy and love. Know that you can always draw this energy from your source or well and that this energy is limitless. Then visualize this energy flowing throughout your entire body to revitalize and re-energize it. Visualize this energy bringing light to any areas of darkness anywhere in your body or mind. Feel the certainty that you are your own source of unlimited healing. Moontime blessings!

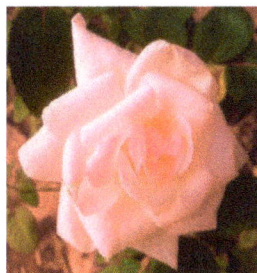

SHE DANCES WITH *the* SONG *of* HER MOON
For Avra's Menarche

This was inspired by my daughter Avra as she flowed into her menarche one sunny summer day.

She awakes to the surprise. She is new and alive. Her body has entered the flow of the Goddess and she is emerging into the web of oneness with all wembyn. She is flowing into the stream of her femininity and is becoming a wombyn. She is still but a child, but will soon awaken to the joys, wonders and mysteries of a wombyn's life.

The birth of beauty, the power of her body to give the gift of life. Now becoming a channel of Goddess love, you can cross the psychic veil each month and wander through the void to discover what treasures are buried there to be retrieved and brought back into the world that you create.

Go now and visit the Goddess within each month. Let your blood flow onto the earth-to nurture, to share her power, her strength. Let your healing flow as the essence of your fertility flows, from within to without. You can now find the answers to heal yourself. Listen to your body as it tells you what it needs. Let it tell you how you can maintain your balance and harmony.

You now have a new sister-the moon. She'll remind you of your cycles of dark and light, your time to shine and your time to be still and quiet. Honor your sister moon, our Mother Earth-all part of the light of creation within and without. Welcome!

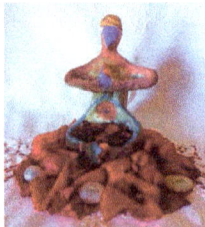

Sun	Mon	Tue	Wed	Thu	Fri	Sat

IDEAS and SUGGESTIONS to FOLLOW

1. Journal - uncensored thoughts, feelings, reactions to this month's moontime.

_____
_____
_____
_____
_____

2. Dreams and Visions - messages from the unconscious, from your Goddess self.

_____
_____
_____
_____
_____

3. Special self-nurturing reminders - things to do for yourself during your moontime, or during the month, to sustain healing.

_____
_____
_____
_____
_____

4. Preparations needed to create a harmonious moontime - i.e., reminders for child care, appointments to make or cancel, items to purchase, candles to have for a bath.

_____
_____
_____
_____
_____

5. Reminders for food and diet- when to change or eliminate certain foods, take supplements, herbs to have on hand, things to do that release stress.

_____

_____

_____

_____

_____

6. What old beliefs have been uncovered, need to be eliminated or changed?

_____

_____

_____

_____

_____

7. Reminders of activities that will create a harmonious moontime - make an appointment for a massage, walk in nature, get extra sleep, and listen to music that you love.

_____

_____

_____

_____

_____

8. What did your last moontime reveal that will help make the next one more spiritual or bring you closer to your sacred self?

_____

_____

_____

_____

_____

9. Create your own ritual, draw or paint your feelings and/or dreams.

_____

_____

_____

_____

_____

FOCUS #2
OUR BODY IMAGE

2nd month-Changing Bodies

The next place to explore is your body.

Now that you are flowing monthly, there are other changes that usually happen. Bodies begin to change. Breasts develop, sexual hormones start to flow and the dance of partnership often kicks in.

These body changes introduce young girls into the world of sexual attraction, limitations, unwanted attractions, female competition, likes, dislikes, gender preference, and many judgments fed by media, peers and even family members. There is often a struggle to find acceptance in your body that evolves after menarche or you may delight in the changes if it finds attraction from the outer world. Coping with these changes can be a challenge and more often than not there isn't a healthy avenue to express what you feel.

If a young girl hasn't been taught about the sacredness of her body and emerging wombynhood, she often embraces the mundane beliefs from her peers. Those beliefs bring her into the world of sexual dances and competition, using her body to attract while emulating what media images hold in high esteem which often lacks respect. Everyone wants the *perfect* looking body that the media and fashion industry has told us is perfect.

It is so easy for a wombyn to get caught up in that illusion and carry that with her throughout her life. It creates struggle, weight issues, dissatisfaction with one's body, dysfunctional obsessions, and often emotional turmoil. Is it possible that these thoughts and feelings create the foundation for disharmony or discomforts during one's moontime?

What if your changing body doesn't resemble those contrived images? What if your body isn't thin or tall or beautiful? Does that mean you aren't perfect? Are those images the only reflection of beauty?

Or is there another lens that you can look through? The one that says your body is your temple. It is the corporal home of your spirit and in that light it is always wonderful and blessed. Maybe if you look through the lens that says your body, no matter who she develops into, is really the recipient of love given to you by your inner Goddess and she now has the power to create life. Your changing body is something to be respected, loved and cared for. Loving your temple, a vessel for Divine Feminine energy, is a root that helps your soul to feel at peace with herself. Loving your temple is knowing that you have the respect for yourself that you want others to have for you.

Do you love your temple?

Do you feed your body healthy food and keep her clean, exercise her regularly, adorn her with beauty, treat her with respect and dignity and demand that others do that too?

Have you ever tried yoga, tai chi, been massaged, gone dancing? Do you know how to use herbs and holistic modalities for healing? Does she meditate?

Do you listen to the voice of pain and seek solutions or quiet that voice with medications or substances?

If you abuse your body, if you let others abuse it, you close off to that Divine voice within and lose the opportunity to allow the Sacred wisdom in. If you don't love your body, listen more carefully to why, and reverse what can be reversed and accept what can be accepted. What will it take for you to love your body? If you don't love your body, how can you love you?
Your temple is Sacred and a gift of the Divine. Please treat her with dignity and love.

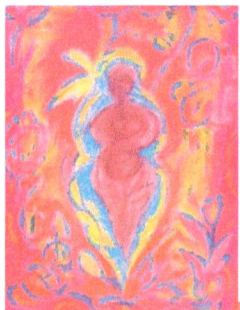

Sun	Mon	Tue	Wed	Thu	Fri	Sat

IDEAS and SUGGESTIONS to FOLLOW

1. Journal - uncensored thoughts, feelings, reactions to this month's moontime.

_____

_____

_____

_____

_____

2. Dreams and Visions - messages from the unconscious, from your Goddess self.

_____

_____

_____

_____

_____

3. Special self-nurturing reminders - things to do for yourself during your moontime, or during the month, to sustain healing.

_____

_____

_____

_____

_____

4. Preparations needed to create a harmonious moontime - i.e., reminders for child care, appointments to make or cancel, items to purchase, candles to have for a bath.

_____

_____

_____

_____

_____

5. Reminders for food and diet- when to change or eliminate certain foods, take supplements, herbs to have on hand, things to do that release stress.

_____
_____
_____
_____
_____

6. What old beliefs have been uncovered, need to be eliminated or changed?

_____
_____
_____
_____
_____

7. Reminders of activities that will create a harmonious moontime - make an appointment for a massage, walk in nature, get extra sleep, and listen to music that you love.

_____
_____
_____
_____
_____

8. What did your last moontime reveal that will help make the next one more spiritual or bring you closer to your sacred self?

_____
_____
_____
_____
_____

9. Create your own ritual, draw or paint your feelings and/or dreams.

_____
_____
_____
_____
_____

FOCUS #3
FEMALE SELF-IMAGE

3rd month-What is Our Feminine Self?

Who are you as a wombyn? Today we are many things, but we are still the life givers of the planet. We bring life into being. We create new life either through our children or we channel creative energy to bring new life through our ideas and talents. We wembyn weave the web of life and keep it going. Our blood is Sacred because it is the holy essence from where life originates. It is the blood that flows without killing. It is the 'heavenly waters,' our moon flower, our wise blood.

Many wembyn inherently like to nurture, heal and love. Some of us have been taught to deny or shut down that part of our nature. That denial can create pain, both physical and emotional. We are often taught to ignore our desire to unconditionally love. We learn to hold back and to protect our hearts. Shutting down our love clogs our beings, it blocks our flow, and what blocks our flow creates disharmony. What creates disharmony leads to pain.

Yet other wembyn allow their inner Hindu Goddess 'Durga' strength to surface, their 'take charge' power. Sometimes it leads to a more male shade of dominance, sometimes it just gets things done. If this assertive strength is used for assuring life survives and wembyn sound louder and stronger voices, they have a better chance to have more control over their destinies. Life has a better chance of surviving. It unblocks their energy, it allows their flows to flow.

Maybe it's time to unclog, open up and rejoice in the essence of your true femininity? Not the model that magazines want you to adopt, but what it truly means to be a wombyn. Not the model that the corporate, male dominated world has conditioned you to believe is the real wombyn either.

Maybe it's time to recognize and remember what your true nature is? Maybe it's time to empower that true nature, the part that supports and gives life? That part that attunes with moontime energy, trusts her intuition, feels confident that her knowing is divine, that she has the capability to heal and manifest these healings for herself, her family and the planet? Maybe…

It is important that every wombyn remembers that her moontime is a gift. Men don't have a physical monthly guidepost to remind them to slow down, look around inside, check in and see what needs to change, be fixed or cleansed. Men keep going until illness or crisis force them to do that, but a wombyn has the opportunity to *retreat* from the outer world and get closer to the Divine when your blood flows each month. Men may strive through years of discipline and spiritual practice to try and achieve connections with their inner worlds. Wembyn can open up to these connections monthly. Wembyn can heal.

Many of the great religions of the world have been controlled and designed by male consciousness. They have designed life so that menstruation is considered to be a time when a wombyn is made to feel dirty and ashamed, often banished for fear of contamination. Yet the real fear, conscious or unconscious, is that a wombyn would be more spiritually powerful and take their power and control away from them. Then they wouldn't be able to dominate and control not just wembyn, but life itself.

Since they can't 'burn us at the stake' anymore, at least not in the Western world, wembyn aren't as terrified into submission as in the past. Still there are corporate, male-dominated power structures that control our daily rhythms and feminine rhythms. They deny the rhythm of the Feminine and ignore the valuable connection that this rhythm has to a wombyn and Mother Earth.

They have turned to ruthlessly dominating and destroying nature instead. Their greed and ignorance supersedes their respect for nature's gifts and beauty. Global threats like climate change and fracking are out of control. Will we be able to rebalance the rhythms of the natural world and eliminate these dangers to Mother Earth? To life itself?

We can't let it continue. Our survival and all life depend on it. Perhaps it is up to wembyn to lead the way back into harmony with nature, by going forward, and asserting our true nature. That essence of wombyn that in not just our sexual or procreative nature, but our Sacred nature as well. Perhaps it is by returning to harmony with our *feminine essence* that we will lead the way to return to a global harmony with nature, mother Gaia and all life itself. Is it not all connected?

It is an important global direction that we remember our feminine essence. Personal, feminine and planetary harmony is linked to this reconnection with the wisdom your moontime. Finding one's moontime harmony is a wonderful place for a wombyn to start in order to reclaim her feminine essence and female self. If you return to the essence of your Sacred Feminine self, your feminine self-image will remember that it is really life giving and divine. Please find, remember and become familiar with your Divine Feminine connection. Listen to her wisdom during your moontime! Trust your moontime truths.

What is your feminine self-image? Is she Sacred and Divine?

What aspect of being feminine gives you the most pleasure, makes you feel the most whole?

What emotions describe your feminine self-image?

Does your feminine self need healing? What would she look like when you are healed?

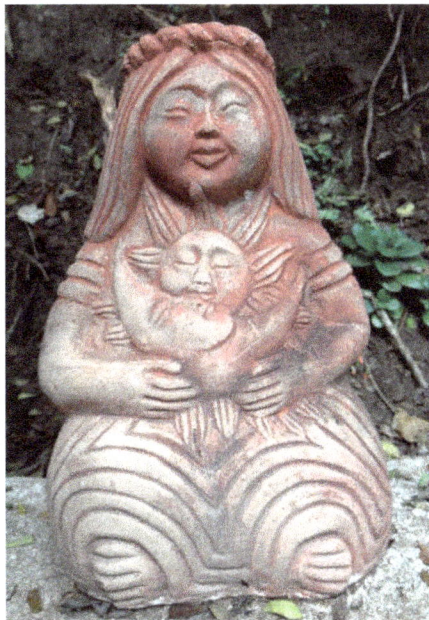

Use this page for notes and play.

Use this page for notes and play.

Sun	Mon	Tue	Wed	Thu	Fri	Sat

IDEAS and SUGGESTIONS to FOLLOW

1. Journal - uncensored thoughts, feelings, reactions to this month's moontime.

_____

_____

_____

_____

_____

2. Dreams and Visions - messages from the unconscious, from your Goddess self.

_____

_____

_____

_____

_____

3. Special self-nurturing reminders - things to do for yourself during your moontime, or during the month, to sustain healing.

_____

_____

_____

_____

_____

4. Preparations needed to create a harmonious moontime - i.e., reminders for child care, appointments to make or cancel, items to purchase, candles to have for a bath.

_____

_____

_____

_____

_____

5. Reminders for food and diet - when to change or eliminate certain foods, take supplements, herbs to have on hand, things to do that release stress.

_____

_____

_____

_____

_____

6. What old beliefs have been uncovered, need to be eliminated or changed?

_____

_____

_____

_____

_____

7. Reminders of activities that will create a harmonious moontime - make an appointment for a massage, walk in nature, get extra sleep, and listen to music that you love.

_____

_____

_____

_____

_____

8. What did your last moontime reveal that will help make the next one more spiritual or bring you closer to your sacred self?

_____

_____

_____

_____

9. Create your own ritual, draw or paint your feelings and/or dreams.

_____

_____

_____

_____

FOCUS #4
SEXUALITY

4th month-What are Your Feelings, Fears, Attitudes Towards Sexuality?

The power to create life originates in one's sexuality. This could be the actual bringing forth of another being or the use of this creative energy to bring forth new ideas or projects. Our sexual rhythms wax and wane with our moontime rhythms. Are you familiar with tantric rituals and that sexuality can create bridges to the Divine?

Sexuality is a charged and vital aspect of our lives. We might like it or not. We might have gender confusion or not. We might use our bodies to attract it or not. We might dress sexy or be embarrassed and avoid dressing sexy. It's with us from our menarche in varying ways and degrees.

But did you know that your sexuality could also be used to heal? Are you aware of the sacred power that sexual energy is capable of generating? Did you know that it has this power? You have this power to use to create bridges to the Divine? Are you familiar with tantric rituals that use sexuality to reach higher levels of awareness?

How are you connected to your sexual expression? Is it an expression of your vital life force, your Shakti nature? Of your heart? Is it satisfying? Ecstatic? Are you connected to your sacred sexual spirit and its power to create life and love? Or does it scare you and make you feel uncomfortable or ashamed? Does sexual intimacy frighten you? Do you feel like an object used and then discarded? Can you express your needs and reactions to your partners? How do you use your sexual power? Is it working?

A huge global problem is the existence of sexual abuse and sexual slavery. Fortunately, there are many avenues of help to assist with healing if you have been sexually abused. There are many books, therapists and outlets to help you uncover the depth and details of your abuse. If you have been abused and want to heal, the buried scars might have to be uncovered. If you have been a victim, you will probably want to find a way to release the traumas so you can unblock the fears, frustrations, anger and pain that have resulted from these horrors. Sexual traumas often create moontime disharmony and pain. They probably need to be released before you can move into a healthy space of moontime harmony and sacred sexuality-a sexuality that includes the heart not just the body. This is the path to sexual healing and moontime wholeness.

Today, the complexity of gender identity has created an even bigger picture of sexuality. If you are challenged by not fitting into the norm, I urge you to find the support that you need so you can be clear and own who you are. Be kind and loving to yourself so that you can be kind and loving to another person. Be gentle with yourself as you explore this most intimate of expressions. Know that you are a Divine being and that this part of you is Divine too.

What is your feeling about your sexuality? Can you make a connection to your moontime?

What would you want your sexual experiences to be like?

What would sacred sexuality look like to you? Would that create moontime harmony too?

If you haven't found healing for sexual trauma, when will you begin and where will you go to find it? If your moontime is painful, might healing these traumas heal your moontime pain?

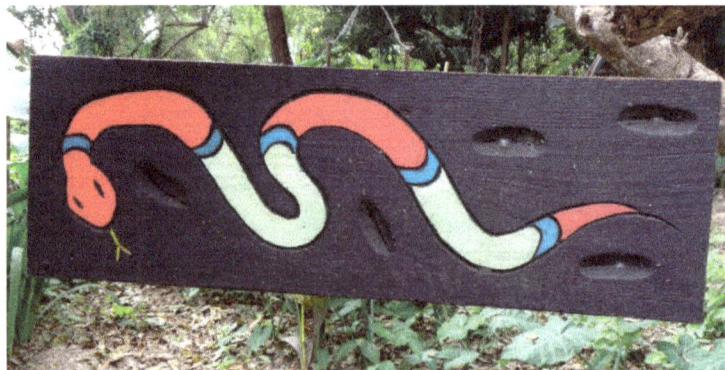

Sun	Mon	Tue	Wed	Thu	Fri	Sat

IDEAS and SUGGESTIONS to FOLLOW

1. Journal - uncensored thoughts, feelings, reactions to this month's moontime.

_____
_____
_____
_____
_____

2. Dreams and Visions - messages from the unconscious, from your Goddess self.

_____
_____
_____
_____
_____

3. Special self-nurturing reminders - things to do for yourself during your moontime, or during the month, to sustain healing.

_____
_____
_____
_____
_____

4. Preparations needed to create a harmonious moontime - i.e., reminders for child care, appointments to make or cancel, items to purchase, candles to have for a bath.

_____
_____
_____
_____
_____

5. Reminders for food and diet - when to change or eliminate certain foods, take supplements, herbs to have on hand, things to do that release stress.

_____

_____

_____

_____

_____

6. What old beliefs have been uncovered, need to be eliminated or changed?

_____

_____

_____

_____

_____

7. Reminders of activities that will create a harmonious moontime - make an appointment for a massage, walk in nature, get extra sleep, and listen to music that you love.

_____

_____

_____

_____

_____

8. What did your last moontime reveal that will help make the next one more spiritual or bring you closer to your sacred self?

_____

_____

_____

_____

_____

9. Create your own ritual, draw or paint your feelings and/or dreams.

_____

_____

_____

_____

_____

FOCUS #5
CREATION and CREATIVITY

5th month-Are You Using Your Blood to Create New Life?

You are a wombyn. You have the ability and the power to bring forth life. You have the power to create life from your womb, but you also have the power to transform the intuitive, the creative and the unconscious and bring these into form and physical reality too. You can communicate with the Divine and the Sacred. You can bring these experiences into life.

The most obvious expression of this power to create life is the birthing of our children- the legacy of life and the future of the survival of the human race. Our bodies have the capacity to transform the nourishment that we feed them into fully-formed human beings. What a miraculous power we have!

Yet this transformative power is not only available for the purpose of maintaining human-kind, it is also available for the birthing of the creative expression of our spirits. It is part of our nature to be able to transform the inner into the outer. It is part of our nature to flow with our feelings, thoughts and inspirations and bring them out into expression. We can be artists, writers, singers, dancers, musicians, mothers, healers, caregivers, actresses, lawyers, politicians, teachers, and more as an expression of our Goddess-given birthright to create. We can be vessels of the transformation of spirit into matter and form.

Just as the energy of the earth transforms the separate elements and weaves them into the physical world; just as the earth has her cycles of light and dark, hot and cold, day and night, life and death; just as the earth destroys and rebuilds; so does a wombyn pass through these same cycles each month. Just as the moon changes from light to dark and back to light again, wembyn have a connection to these rhythms that follow and imitate the cycles and seasons of the earth and the moon. When you become conscious of the rhythms of your feminine life force and attune your *self* to this energy, then you enter into the flow with your feminine creativity. You can express the essence of your feminine power. This can take the direction to give life via a child or through your special brand of creativity.

When you are in harmony with your moontime, your flow will be an inspiration. When you are flowing with your creativity it opens your heart and heals.

Do you flow somewhere where you can be prepared with what you need in order to be creative?

What can you do to allow your creativity to flow?

Have you prepared your moonlodge with the materials for creative expression?

Do you have paints, sketch book, music, a craft, whatever you need to be creative accessible?

Have you tried a new creative expression that was inspired by your moontime?

Have you tried to listen to the voice of your inner Goddess and let her be your muse?

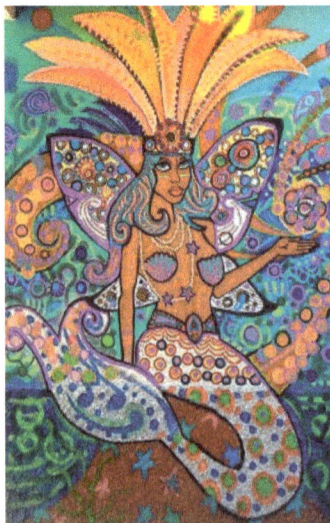

Sun	Mon	Tue	Wed	Thu	Fri	Sat

IDEAS and SUGGESTIONS to FOLLOW

1. Journal - uncensored thoughts, feelings, reactions to this month's moontime.

_____

_____

_____

_____

_____

2. Dreams and Visions - messages from the unconscious, from your Goddess self.

_____

_____

_____

_____

_____

3. Special self-nurturing reminders - things to do for yourself during your moontime, or during the month, to sustain healing.

_____

_____

_____

_____

_____

4. Preparations needed to create a harmonious moontime - i.e., reminders for child care, appointments to make or cancel, items to purchase, candles to have for a bath.

_____

_____

_____

_____

_____

5. Reminders for food and diet - when to change or eliminate certain foods, take supplements, herbs to have on hand, things to do that release stress.

_____

_____

_____

_____

_____

6. What old beliefs have been uncovered, need to be eliminated or changed?

_____

_____

_____

_____

_____

7. Reminders of activities that will create a harmonious moontime - make an appointment for a massage, walk in nature, get extra sleep, and listen to music that you love.

_____

_____

_____

_____

_____

8. What did your last moontime reveal that will help make the next one more spiritual or bring you closer to your sacred self?

_____

_____

_____

_____

_____

9. Create your own ritual, draw or paint your feelings and/or dreams.

_____

_____

_____

_____

_____

Focus #6
Psychic Attunement

6ᵗʰ month-How Sharp is Your Psychic Radar?

The veil thins between the conscious and the unconscious every month during your moontime. That means that you have the opportunity to be more psychically aware and intuitive. A wombyn needs to dream, take time to listen to her body and allow her flow to nurture and heal. When she can slow down and attune to her sacred, inner space; the doorway to the Divine opens and she can journey into the Void. It is there, in the Void, where you can commune with the Goddess within, connect to your higher, Sacred Self. It is in that Sacred void that you can access solutions, visions, creative decisions, and healing wisdom that can be brought back and out into your reality and daily life. This ability is your innate potential when you honor and respect your moontime

So how do you attune to the psychic changes that are flowing through you each month? Many wembyn need to create an environment that supports this energy in order to access that part of their psychic self. You probably need to be alone because it is when you are in the quiet stillness of your own inner world and thoughts that your inner and intuitive knowing will flow more easily.

Going within might take the form of prayer, meditation, resting, singing, dancing, writing, reading, drawing, or taking a walk in nature. Whatever you are drawn to do will be the right activity for you so that you can listen to what your inner world wants to tell you. By shutting out the interferences and noise of the outer world, you can freely drift and dream within and *hear* what your inner world wants you to hear. Moontimes offer you the opportunity to flow where your spirit needs you to flow. It is your inner life or darkness giving birth to your outer life and light. It is the void or emptiness giving voice to what needs to be heard.

A wombyn who has a busy or active life would benefit by finding and taking the time to honor this need. Isn't it better to take this time consciously instead of having your body make you take that time by creating cramps and pains that then force you to take this time out? It is so valuable to honor this amazing and natural aspect of your moontime rhythm, this intuitive component that brings you closer to the Divine. It is so healing to flow with this gift rather than ignoring or fighting against her.

Have you ever heard or felt what your moontime *self* has spoken to you as she guided you with her knowledge?

Did she show you how to create a more harmonious moontime, heal an imbalance or solve a problem?

Did you feel this knowing in your heart and soul?

What might you need to do so that you can listen and hear your intuitive voice?

Can you slow down, listen to the quiet and hear the subtle and soft voice of the Divine within?

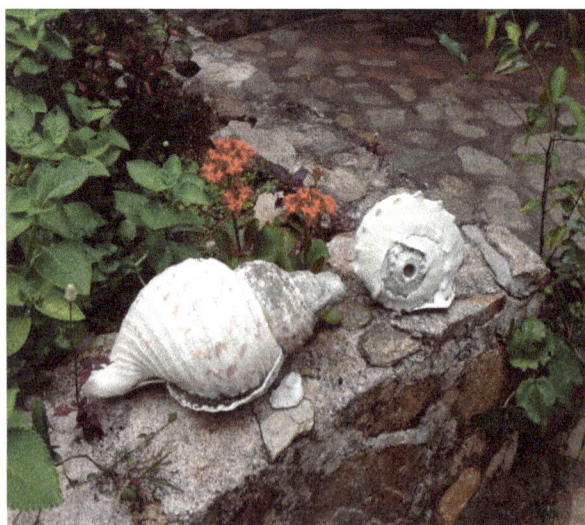

Sun	Mon	Tue	Wed	Thu	Fri	Sat

Ideas and SUGGESTIONS to FOLLOW

1. Journal - uncensored thoughts, feelings, reactions to this month's moontime.

_____

_____

_____

_____

_____

2. Dreams and Visions - messages from the unconscious, from your Goddess self.

_____

_____

_____

_____

_____

3. Special self-nurturing reminders - things to do for yourself during your moontime, or during the month, to sustain healing.

_____

_____

_____

_____

_____

4. Preparations needed to create a harmonious moontime - i.e., reminders for child care, appointments to make or cancel, items to purchase, candles to have for a bath.

_____

_____

_____

_____

_____

5. Reminders for food and diet - when to change or eliminate certain foods, take supplements, herbs to have on hand, things to do that release stress.

_____

_____

_____

_____

_____

6. What old beliefs have been uncovered, need to be eliminated or changed?

_____

_____

_____

_____

_____

7. Reminders of activities that will create a harmonious moontime - make an appointment for a massage, walk in nature, get extra sleep, and listen to music that you love.

_____

_____

_____

_____

_____

8. What did your last moontime reveal that will help make the next one more spiritual or bring you closer to your sacred self?

_____

_____

_____

_____

_____

9. Create your own ritual, draw or paint your feelings and/or dreams.

_____

_____

_____

_____

_____

Focus #7

Rituals

7th month-Creating Meaningful Rituals

How can you make your moontimes sacred? How do you enter into harmony with your flow? How do you create a ritual, each month, to honor the entrance into the domain of the Goddess?

What are rituals? What do they do? Why are they helpful?

Simply, rituals are ways of marking and acknowledging the existence of a special event or moment in one's life. They can be collective, traditional events or original and self-created moments that have meaning to you. Often situations that require a ritual start with an opening for the ritual, the ritual itself and a closing gesture-a beginning, middle and an end.

The actual moment that starts your moontime is often a surprise, but you begin to move into your moontime space a few days before you begin to flow. There's often a change of mood accompanied by specific physical changes. Instead of being reactive or overwhelmed by these changes, it helps to mark your transition into your moontime space with a ritual. By punctuating the change with a conscious activity that makes you feel good, you can honor and enter the space you are moving into with positive feelings.

As you begin to realize that you are entering into your moontime cave, lodge or temple, it may help you to feel more attuned to your energetic changes if you create another ritual. Perhaps an altar with red flowers, set out some red crystals or have an activity prepared that you know will help you with this attunement. Maybe lighting some incense made from red flowers, surround yourself with red candles or smudging with sage. Beginning to write in a red moontime journal can help bring your awareness into the present moment.

Once your flow begins your rituals may change. You might be drawn to create a mandala, listen to music that moves you, read poetry that speaks to you, lay dreaming while covered with a warm and cozy red blanket or prepare meals made from red foods. These are just some examples of rituals that you can prepare for and look forward to each moontime. They can always change, as your needs change. Ideally you'll be inspired to prepare what works for you.

Then, when you are emerging from your moonlodge and ready to re-enter life again, you can mark that with another ritual. A ritual that evokes gratitude, a prayer and thanks to the Goddess within, a gift you have created, or made that will offer thanks to the wisdom, lessons, strength, or healings that were part of that month's flow. Perhaps you can create a ritual of blessings to share with the world or people you live with.

Rituals help focus the energy or give attention to something that needs to be looked at or remembered. They can be simple as well as avenues for your creativity. They are important because they remind you of something that might get lost or forgotten. They bring light into the darkness.

Did you use any rituals for your moontime? What were they?

Have you created any new ones?

How do your rituals enhance your moontime experience?

Do your rituals help you to create moontime order out of chaos, help you to follow your cycles?

Have your rituals helped you to tune into your moontime awareness with greater clarity?

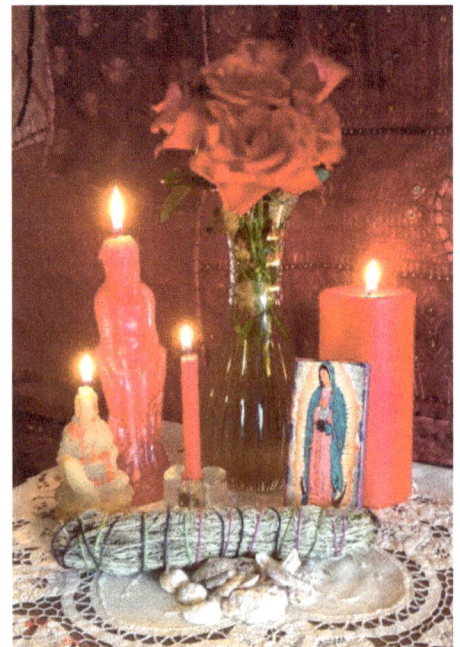

Sun	Mon	Tue	Wed	Thu	Fri	Sat

IDEAS and SUGGESTIONS to FOLLOW

1. Journal - uncensored thoughts, feelings, reactions to this month's moontime.

_____
_____
_____
_____
_____

2. Dreams and Visions - messages from the unconscious, from your Goddess self.

_____
_____
_____
_____
_____

3. Special self-nurturing reminders - things to do for yourself during your moontime, or during the month, to sustain healing.

_____
_____
_____
_____
_____

4. Preparations needed to create a harmonious moontime - i.e., reminders for child care, appointments to make or cancel, items to purchase, candles to have for a bath.

_____
_____
_____
_____
_____

5. Reminders for food and diet - when to change or eliminate certain foods, take supplements, herbs to have on hand, things to do that release stress.

_____
_____
_____
_____
_____

6. What old beliefs have been uncovered, need to be eliminated or changed?

_____
_____
_____
_____
_____

7. Reminders of activities that will create a harmonious moontime - make an appointment for a massage, walk in nature, get extra sleep, and listen to music that you love.

_____
_____
_____
_____
_____

8. What did your last moontime reveal that will help make the next one more spiritual or bring you closer to your sacred self?

_____
_____
_____
_____
_____

9. Create your own ritual, draw or paint your feelings and/or dreams.

_____
_____
_____
_____
_____

FOCUS #8

PAIN

8th month-Where Does Your Moontime Pain Come From?

If your moontime is accompanied by pain, either physical or emotional or both, here are some questions you might ask yourself.

Do you love your moontime? Why not?

What don't you love about your monthly flow?

What do you love about being a wombyn? What don't you love about being a wombyn?

Do you love your body? Your sexuality?

How do you feel about men, the business world you may work in, male based religions that dominant and control?

If you are gay or transgender, how does your monthly menstrual cycle affect you and your identity?

Have you ever closely looked at, touched, felt, and smelled your menstrual blood? Or are you ashamed or embarrassed by your blood?

Do you ever let your blood flow out onto Mother Earth? Have you sat and communed with Her during your moontime?

Do you fear or dread the arrival of your period?

Is your identity as a wombyn linked to your mothering, sexuality, job, creativity, role in your family, attention from men?

Do you envy men because they don't have a monthly period?

Is your moontime pleasurable or painful?

Have you made an attempt to lessen or eliminate your pain by nurturing yourself before or during your moontime? What would that nurturing look like? Did it help?

It has been observed that we create pain from the top down, from the inner to the outer. What I mean is that physical discomfort and pain (with the exception of surgery, accidents, childbirth for some) may be the result of spiritual disharmony that originates in our spirit or emotional worlds and eventually filters down into our physical world in the form of pain. The pain is then a reflection of an imbalance and a lack of harmony within one's being. It is possible to numb the pain when need be, but to truly eliminate it and return to a state of harmony, one must uncover and release the sources of blockages that create the pain. And those blockages can take many forms.

They can come from untrue or negative beliefs, poor diet, built-up stress, lack of exercise, emotional traumas that were never healed; just to name just a few.

Physical situations often result from emotional scars and hurts that get lodged in one's cells unconsciously. Pain becomes the body's way to attract attention to these scars. Frequently this pain has roots in old and unresolved hurts. Often it is the result of some part of us that was unloved. Pain is often your body's way of saying, "pay attention to me I need to be mended and cared for."

Menstrual pain often begins with our menarche or first period. How many of us experienced our first moontime as a celebration into the world of life-giving wombynhood energy? How many of us enjoyed the pleasure of knowing that we were becoming fully whole, sexually creative flowers that could express the feminine flow of energy of creation? How many of us entered this new realm with joy and excitement?

All too often our scars originated with the first drop of our blood. The negative programming took root easily, because pain was what your mother, sister, friend, or an aunt experienced. What could have been joyful is far too often experienced with pain and fear. This pain and fear then gets attached to the very core of our feminine nature and might even increase over time.

Even our fathers may have retreated from us once we became a menstruating wombyn. Yes they still loved us, but were afraid to touch or be affectionate with the now sexual girl/wombyn. And a confused young mind often interprets this as her fault even though she never did anything but grow breasts and hips and become sexually alluring. Or worse yet, touching was continued in these new places on our body without respect for our feelings. Our spiritual female, or our sense of ourselves as divine creators of life, is rarely given support or acknowledgment.

The unexpressed sadness that many adolescent girls experience when one or both parents pull away emotionally after the beginning of menarche is a potential source of pain that may reoccur every month. The emotional pain with the loss of your father's (male) love, the emotional pain of leaving the loving security of childhood, the pain of entering into the isolation and abandonment of adolescent femininity, the painful confusion when the body changes and becomes the focus for success or disapproval; all become sources for disharmony that may surface in menstrual physical or emotional pain later in life.

There can be pain surrounding emerging and conflicting sexual desires and attitudes. A girl might have to choose between Madonna or whore, slut or good girl. One choice might be connected with the loss of heartfelt love from the people who are near to her and yet the other choice would ask her to deny what her own needs may be or peer popularity. Then the transgender, gay, bisexual young female runs up against a whole other set of conflicts when emerging into the society she lives in. All this because our blood begins to flow. No wonder our ovaries and uterus are in pain!

Pain has become a way of life for many wembyn. Emotional and physical pain are almost accepted as the norm, especially when connected to our moontime. We live fast-paced lives, work in cold, unemotional business worlds and deal with people who are too busy to stop or care. We experience alienation from our spirits and the spirit of nature as we live and work in structures that keep us separate from Mother Earth. We are estranged from the living, breathing earth that gives us her unconditional love. We suffer from repressed creativity and low self-esteem. We may harbor frustration resulting from male dominance and inequality, cope with pollution, electromagnetic interferences, eat denatured food, live rhythms that lack attunement with the cycles of the Earth and the Moon. Are these not fertile ground for pain?

The question is how can we transform our painful moontimes into sacred, blessed experiences? How can we change the darkness of pain into the light of joy?

The beginning is often the most needed place to clear. Try returning to the moment of your menarche. Remember how you experienced it, the feelings, your thoughts, and emotions. What people might have said to you. And then if it wasn't a beautiful experience, recreate it the way you would have wanted it to be. Visualize a recreation. Who would you have wanted to share that time with? What ceremonies and celebrations might you have wanted to take place? What rituals would you have wanted to be taught that you could reenact each month?

Do this during your moontime, let your mind wander and dream the visions of a healthier and more aware menarche. It was your special moment and it should have been respected, honored and celebrated. Recreate your initiation into the *blood mysteries* of the feminine energy of life the way you needed it to be.

Ask your next moontime why the pain is there. Talk to the pain, sadness, tension, either silently or out loud. Ask it where it came from, what lessons it is trying to teach you and what changes you need to make to return to balance and harmony. Instead of hating the pain, try to honor it as a teacher. Let the pain talk and listen.

Another technique is to write a letter to your pain. Speak to it and then listen for its answers and write down the pain's reply. Release the answers from your psyche in a letter, a drawing, a song, a poem, or a painting.

Be still and listen, meditate on the answers, take a walk in nature and let the natural world bring you her answers. Take a bath with sweet smelling salts, bleed onto the earth and ask Mother Earth for the clarity you need.

Once you have opened up to your pain, listen to its answers, then empower them. Remember that you are cleaning out the old and replacing it with something new. Touch the pain, send love to the unloved, hurting places. Send forgiveness to the people or situations that consciously or unconsciously caused you pain. Release and let go and replace the loss with positive affirmations, thoughts and actions that move you into health and harmony. Write them down and repeat them. Make the changes that need to be made and know that your inner, Goddess Self is guiding you. When you replace the pain and hurt with positive images, you send messages to your unconscious to help you release the old patterns and programs so that you can replace them with positive, healing ones. Use your power as a wombyn to create by creating a new, loving, beautiful, happy, radiant, alive, painless moontime image. You are in control and you can heal yourself.

Remember to start slowly and gently. Make a list of your needed changes. Choose just one or a few per month to work on. Don't pressure yourself. Start with the ones that you will be the most successful with. Give changes times to work. Don't get discouraged and be patient. Like a flower that needs protection, nurturing and care, let your changes unfold safely and at their own pace.

Pray to the Goddess for light, strength and guidance. She is you and within you and always there.

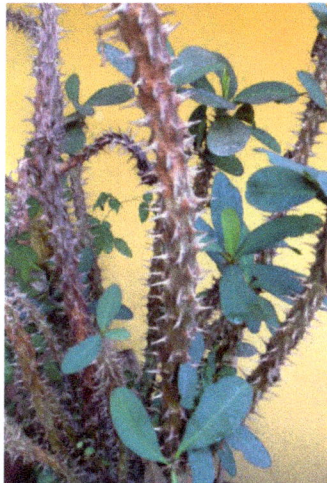

Use this page for notes and play.

Use this page for notes and play.

Sun	Mon	Tue	Wed	Thu	Fri	Sat

IDEAS and SUGGESTIONS to FOLLOW

1. Journal - uncensored thoughts, feelings, reactions to this month's moontime.

_____
_____
_____
_____
_____

2. Dreams and Visions - messages from the unconscious, from your Goddess self.

_____
_____
_____
_____
_____

3. Special self-nurturing reminders - things to do for yourself during your moontime, or during the month, to sustain healing.

_____
_____
_____
_____
_____

4. Preparations needed to create a harmonious moontime - i.e., reminders for child care, appointments to make or cancel, items to purchase, candles to have for a bath.

_____
_____
_____
_____
_____

5. Reminders for food and diet - when to change or eliminate certain foods, take supplements, herbs to have on hand, things to do that release stress.

_____

_____

_____

_____

_____

6. What old beliefs have been uncovered, need to be eliminated or changed?

_____

_____

_____

_____

_____

7. Reminders of activities that will create a harmonious moontime - make an appointment for a massage, walk in nature, get extra sleep, and listen to music that you love.

_____

_____

_____

_____

_____

8. What did your last moontime reveal that will help make the next one more spiritual or bring you closer to your sacred self?

_____

_____

_____

_____

_____

9. Create your own ritual, draw or paint your feelings and/or dreams.

_____

_____

_____

_____

_____

Focus #9

PMS

9th *month-Pre-Moontime Signals*

This workbook is not designed to address organic problems or solutions for cramps or PMS. There are real and there are biological reasons why a wombyn experiences physical menstrual pain. The pain is real. A professional practitioner can best suggest courses of treatment, but how clever of our bodies to give us indications that we are moving into our moontime! The question is why must it be painful? Or must it? Why is this called a 'syndrome' when menstruation isn't a disease.

What intelligence to have an automatic body *alarm clock* to remind us that it is time to create a protected and harmonious moontime space. How enlightened is one's body and emotions to send out signals that cannot be ignored to remind a wombyn, that soon her flow will be arriving and it is time to get ready.

Only, unfortunately, many of these reminders are uncomfortable, painful and/or inconvenient to the lives of modern wembyn. The signals are troublesome and there usually isn't time to listen to what they may need because modern life hasn't made space for our natural rhythms to be honored.

Today many wembyn suffer with several bodily and emotional miseries during their monthly cycle. They might begin up to two weeks before they start to flow. They might get more intense as they approach their flow and interrupt the wellbeing of their lives, while other wombyn have little or no significant changes and are barely bothered. Some wombyn experience weight gain, acne, headaches, bloating, cramps, backache, craving for sweets, breast tenderness, or heart pounding to name just a few. There might be emotional signals like crying, depression, mood swings, nervous tension, irritability, anxiety, or forgetfulness. Some wembyn suffer severely, others hardly at all. Some believe that hormones are imbalanced, lack of proper nutrition or exercise are to blame.

If you are out of touch with what your body is asking of you, she will find a way to let you know that you are not in harmony with what she needs.

Often there are ways to reduce, if not totally eliminate many, if not all, of the discomforts of such pre-moontime signals. It takes some investigation, some reading and perhaps visits with a holistic health care practitioner to discover what is happening to your body and what types of help you need and what is available. If you go the route of holistic medicine, it might take some trust, patience, time, and confidence that natural remedies work. It might take some tweaking of doses or times of usage.

Lifestyle and diet changes, inclusions of certain vitamins, herbs or minerals, exercising, yoga, tai chi, acupuncture, and massage can all have huge benefits to alleviate or eliminate pre-moontime discomforts.

There are many well-researched and clearly-written books that explain PMS, as well as many qualified healing modalities that offer help to reduce pain and discomfort. A professional can also offer healing possibilities to minimize or eliminate the emotional upheavals associated with hormonal or nutritional changes during your moontime. By becoming aware of your personal needs, deficiencies or necessary lifestyle changes; you can create a healing program either on your own or with the help of a professional. Pre-moontime signals are not necessarily pains to be escaped, they can be reminders that it is time to get ready for the journey that will unfold in the next few days. If there is pain, maybe something is out of balance. That is your body's way of calling to you and asking for your attention.

Set your intention to create a pain free, emotionally balanced moontime and let your inner wisdom and guidance help you by consciously or serendipitously bringing you the knowledge or person who will help you attain this goal. Research possible causes and possible solutions. Seek out the advice of a professional. You have the power to change this. Listen to your inner guidance and trust.

Some useful statements and affirmations may be:

This month I will....

When I feel my PMS starting I know it is time to....

I don't have to suffer PMS anymore because now I can....

My moontime is my teacher and she will show me what to do when.....

I will examine my diet to see if changes need to be made and make them.

I will explore new avenues like yoga, acupuncture, herbal teas, etc. to help with my PMS.

Next month I will have things in order so I will know what I need to when my PMS...

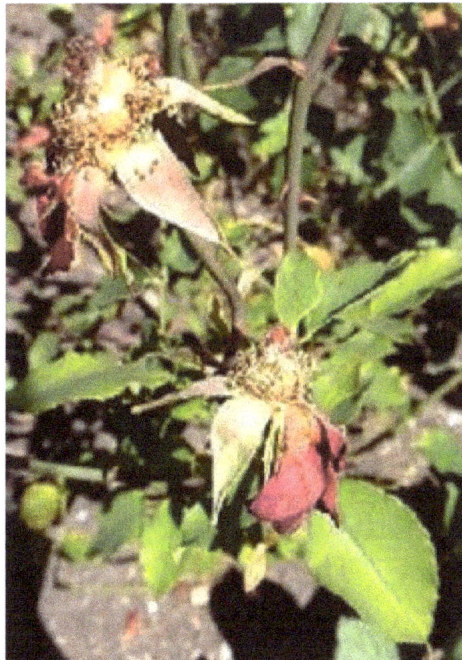

Use this page for notes and play.

Use this page for notes and play.

Sun	Mon	Tue	Wed	Thu	Fri	Sat

IDEAS and SUGGESTIONS to FOLLOW

1. Journal - uncensored thoughts, feelings, reactions to this month's moontime.

_____
_____
_____
_____
_____

2. Dreams and Visions - messages from the unconscious, from your Goddess self.

_____
_____
_____
_____
_____

3. Special self-nurturing reminders - things to do for yourself during your moontime, or during the month, to sustain healing.

_____
_____
_____
_____
_____

4. Preparations needed to create a harmonious moontime - i.e., reminders for child care, appointments to make or cancel, items to purchase, candles to have for a bath.

_____
_____
_____
_____
_____

5. Reminders for food and diet - when to change or eliminate certain foods, take supplements, herbs to have on hand, things to do that release stress.

_____

_____

_____

_____

_____

6. What old beliefs have been uncovered, need to be eliminated or changed?

_____

_____

_____

_____

_____

7. Reminders of activities that will create a harmonious moontime - make an appointment for a massage, walk in nature, get extra sleep, and listen to music that you love.

_____

_____

_____

_____

_____

8. What did your last moontime reveal that will help make the next one more spiritual or bring you closer to your sacred self?

_____

_____

_____

_____

_____

9. Create your own ritual, draw or paint your feelings and/or dreams.

_____

_____

_____

_____

_____

FOCUS #10

SISTER MOON

10th month-We Are Sisters of the Moon

Sister to the Earth Mother Gaia

She reflects the sun's light back to the earth.
She has a light and dark side.
Her light grows in cycles or phases from fullness to emptiness
and back to fullness every twenty eight days.
The moon waxes and wanes from light to dark and back to light again.
She shines silvery streams of light to illuminate earth's shadows and darkness.
She influences the tides of the oceans on the earth
and the tides of emotions within us.
She travels around Gaia Mother Earth every twenty eight days.
The word lunacy comes from lunar or moon.
Lunacy occurs when the energy of the moon illuminates the dark side
Of our psyche or shadows within.
Menstrual, moontime cycles are reflections of
the phases, cycles and energy of the moon.
The Goddess of the Moon is Diana.
She is also the Goddess of Change.

Wembyn are sisters of the moon. She influences our monthly cycle. Just like our sister, we pass through cycles of light and dark. Just like the moon, our emotions wax and wane each month. Just like phases of the moon, our energy waxes and wanes during our moon-time. Our moontimes reflect the light of the moon because they have the power to illuminate our darkness. Wombyn's moontimes are reflections of the phases of the moon.

The moon connects us to our sacred moontime power. When we are in harmony with the energy of the moon, we bleed at the new moon. When we bleed at the new moon, we are ready to receive the seed that might be implanted in our fertile womb at the full moon to begin a new life. When we bleed at the full moon, we become ready to receive the seeds of creation for a new creative life that might surface at the new moon. Wembyn who live together in harmony with the moon often bleed at the same time.

When we are in harmony with our Sister Moon, we receive her power when we bleed. If we are in harmony with the moon, we become vessels and channels of lunar energy. This feminine life-giving energy has the power to nurture and heal with its love. As you bleed, you become a conduit for this energy that flows through you. As you let it flow, like full moon lunar light, it illuminates your darkness and disharmony. This flow can heal as she shines this Divine light into your inner dark spaces.

The word *lunacy* comes from the word *lunar*, meaning moon. It means crazy because emotions often intensify around the full moon. The power that the full moon has is to illuminate and bring to the conscious mind the awareness of your dark side and the shadows of your unconscious mind. These buried fears, worries, doubts, and pains surface into a lighter more conscious clarity. This lunar light reveals what needs cleansing, renewing, or replacing. It is the opportunity when the dark or old can be replaced with the new, lighter and more harmonious thoughts, actions or emotions. Our moontimes follow this lunar cycle. Our moontimes illuminate our dark and old for the purpose of creating and replacing with the new. This is how the power and connection to lunar harmony heals.

The wembyn of the ancient, matriarchal societies knew about their connection to the moon and understood this aspect of their feminine essence. Men respected it and did not fear its power. Modern, and out of touch with nature, societies have become blocked to this knowledge and wisdom. Ancient knowledge that wombyn is a temple for sacred wisdom has been all but forgotten or blocked, and this blockage obstructs our flow. When you don't flow in harmony with the moon and her phases and cycles, it can create blockages that often result in pain, irregularity, and upheavals. Your moontime isn't in harmony.

Since your menstrual cycle is a reflection of the cycles of the moon, it's most helpful to be in harmony with the cycles of the moon to have harmonious moontimes. In order to be in harmony with the moon, you need to be in harmony with the cycles of the light and dark within, as well as without. When a wombyn is in harmony with Sister Moon, she shines her light into your world and you are a conscious vessel for her sacredness. When you flow in harmony with lunar light, you are aware that you wax and wane within your own cycles of light and darkness. When you flow in harmony with the cycles of Sister Moon, the rhythms of your monthly cycle align with hers and become clear. When you flow in harmony, the cycles within your moontime become familiar and your physical, emotional and psychic flows are no longer mysteries.

What a gift to have a sisterly connection who helps to illuminate, like a lunar flashlight, your internal rhythms. This creates balance and harmony. When you flow in alignment with Sister Moon's phases of light and dark, your light and dark phases and hers are connected.

Do you have a calendar that charts the phases of the moon?

Better yet have you looked up in the sky to look at Luna's phases?

Can you connect your phases with Luna's phases, your darkness with hers, your light with hers?

Have you kept track or followed these changes in a journal so you can see and discover your rhythm?

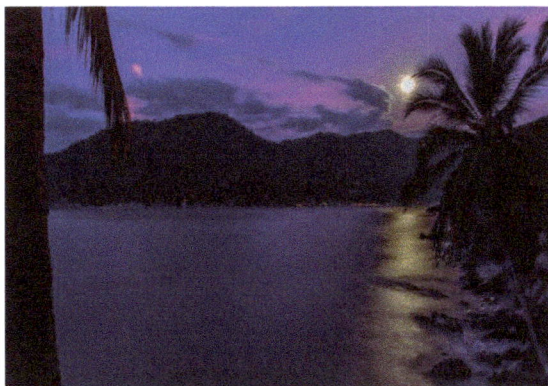

Use this page for notes and play.

Use this page for notes and play.

Sun	Mon	Tue	Wed	Thu	Fri	Sat

Ideas *and* Suggestions *to* Follow

1. Journal - uncensored thoughts, feelings, reactions to this month's moontime.

_____

_____

_____

_____

_____

2. Dreams and Visions - messages from the unconscious, from your Goddess self.

_____

_____

_____

_____

_____

3. Special self-nurturing reminders - things to do for yourself during your moontime, or during the month, to sustain healing.

_____

_____

_____

_____

_____

4. Preparations needed to create a harmonious moontime - i.e., reminders for child care, appointments to make or cancel, items to purchase, candles to have for a bath.

_____

_____

_____

_____

_____

5. Reminders for food and diet - when to change or eliminate certain foods, take supplements, herbs to have on hand, things to do that release stress.

_____

_____

_____

_____

_____

6. What old beliefs have been uncovered, need to be eliminated or changed?

_____

_____

_____

_____

_____

7. Reminders of activities that will create a harmonious moontime - make an appointment for a massage, walk in nature, get extra sleep, and listen to music that you love.

_____

_____

_____

_____

_____

8. What did your last moontime reveal that will help make the next one more spiritual or bring you closer to your sacred self?

_____

_____

_____

_____

9. Create your own ritual, draw or paint your feelings and/or dreams.

_____

_____

_____

_____

Focus #11

The Moontime Medicine Wheel

11th month-Circling Around Your Moontime Medicine Wheel

A wombyn's psychic and intuitive connection to her inner, unconscious world holds the key to creating a harmonious moontime. A wombyn is closer to these inner spaces during her moontime. Attaining balance and harmony on the inside is the foundation for finding balance and harmony during one's moontime. Creating balance and harmony on the inside is the foundation for creating balance and harmony on the outside.

Your moontime often has several phases to her rhythm. Before, during and after the actual flow can vary. And the amount and type of energy you experience changes throughout your flow.

The days that lead up to your flow might be accompanied by irritability, changes in sexual intensity or food cravings. This is your signal that your moontime is soon to arrive.

Once you are in moontime, you might feel a desire to slow down and be alone without any distractions. This is so you can stop and take a look around at what you need to pay attention to and nurture. It is a time for rest and to focus on your needs. It's also a time when a wombyn has the opportunity to descend and flow into the Void to commune with her Goddess within. It is in this *sacred space* that you may be receptive to receiving messages, hearing answers, tapping into your creativity, or taking time to heal.

As a wombyn emerges from the/her void, she travels to a new place along the spiral of her consciousness. There may be a new knowing or shift in perception. This new place will grow and mature in the following months. Honoring this process creates balance. After your moontime stops her flow, you often feel energized, calmer and ready to emerge back into life again.

THE MOONTIME MEDICINE WHEEL

I often experienced my moontime rhythm as following a similar pattern to that of the ritual of the Native American medicine wheel. This process honors the four directions of life and spirit by entering into a sacred circle that honors the four cardinal directions. Each direction-east, south, west, north-reflects a different aspect of the *self* or *soul* and helps it to find clarity on one's journey through life during this earthly existence. Each direction offers a different perspective of how our consciousness grows. Each direction is part of the whole and we need to experience it all to become whole. Like the four seasons of the earth, a wombyn transits through four seasons during our moontime.

Every month a wombyn has the opportunity to travel through all her four directions around her medicine wheel. Knowing this is like traveling with a moontime map that can help to clarify where you are within yourself and where you are going.

In the ritual of the medicine wheel, one enters the sacred circle in the *east*. The east symbolizes the beginning, illumination, birth, springtime. The sun rises in the east, and you enter your moontime space 2-4 days before your flow begins. You enter our moontime in the east. Tensions often arise, your energies may move faster, creativity may increase and often your sexuality might intensify. It is a time to remember that you are approaching your sacred space and it is time to gather what you will need to have a safe, protected and harmonious experience. During this phase of your cycle, your moontime is reminding you to try to pace your responsibilities for the next few days, eliminate what can be left out and prepare to nurture yourself. Whatever will need attention will begin to appear in your mind and/or body. The whispers of the wisdom of your moontime begin to surface.

From the east, in this clockwise circle, you move down to the *south*, the place of youth, noonday, summer, and the physical. Your moontime arrives and the clarity of what needs attention will begin to take shape. It is often the time when you feel the need to slow down, drift and dream. It is during this process of slowing down that allows you the opportunity to discover what is out of balance, what needs clarity, what problems seek solutions, what unresolved issues require attention.

Your thoughts, emotions or bodily reactions heighten. What you have feared, buried or have been too busy to look at will work its way up into your conscious world. If you have avoided confronting something, it may show itself as pain, sadness, anger, or emotional turmoil. Listen to its voice as the issue becomes clearer in the south. If there isn't any major issue craving attention, you may feel the enjoyment of dreaming and drifting, which invites creative inspiration.

Once you have identified what needs attention, your cycle and moontime consciousness move on to the more emotional *west,* called *the dark waters within.* The west holds the setting sun, harvest, teenager, and young adult. It is the season of fall.

In the south you recognized what you needed to see or feel in the physical realm, in the west your emotions may kick in. You understand what situations need attention, solutions or changes your wise moontime wisdom is sending to you. You travel into your void, the place of the unknown. This becomes the time for surrender. It is here that you may experience despair or helplessness. It can be in this phase that you feel the most physical and/or emotional pain and vulnerability. Yet it is also the place of the death of the old, giving up, and letting go of something that no longer works for your life and needs to be left behind. It is the place where you plunge into bottomless valleys. It is here, in the void, where you can search for the source of your pain (parents, abuse, patriarchal beliefs, partners, and work, violating your inner cores) and where the solution will be found. It is here where you can get in touch with your inner Divine, the well of sacred life force, and find answers. This is the garden of the Goddess.

It is in the west that the landscape of your shadow, dark side is revealed. The time to observe where your flow goes and what your unconscious wants to shed light on. A time to welcome the lessons and accept the truths that show you what is not appropriate or needed anymore.

Or you may pass through the void quickly and gently because you've been creating harmony and have been living in a space of balance. Creative inspiration and ideas might surface instead. Each month is different.

When you leave the west, you travel up to the *north,* the place of spirit. The north represents the winter, the wisdom of the elder, death and rebirth. The north will show you what your spirit teachings are for that month. It is here that your inner world begins to reconnect with a sense of peace. You begin to feel like you are being put back together again. The situations or answers are clear, the nurturing has healed you, the rest has renewed you and any visions or changes take hold. Creativity may soar as your energy picks up. *Like a snake skin, the old has been shed and the new born or reborn.* Your inner Goddess has radiated her light, you have communed in her divine temple.

When you move into the north you often feel physically lighter, cleansed, rested, more energetic, stronger, and you begin to feel ready to move out and on with life again. You are ready to re-enter the outer flow of life and do so with a sense of inner harmony. There's a renewed strength and lightness with a desire to manifest the realizations and discoveries that were unveiled to you during your stay in the west.

The sacred space of the moontime continues for a few days after your flow stops. Being aware of this helps you to respect and honor all the feelings and thoughts that flow on after your flow ends. Now you emerge into life stronger, nurtured and energized, ready to resume your daily life and responsibilities. You bring the awareness of changes or healings that you may need to include in your life during the next month. Or you might emerge having created a painting, written a song or poem while you connected and communed with the Sacred and Divine. This moontime circle is over, but the wisdom remains.

Can you follow your moontime seasons? Time and chart them in your journal?

Do you recognize the changes and connect with your moontime phases?

Is there a moment when you recognize your flow's changes? Can you create a ritual to acknowledge them?

Are there moontime patterns that emerge each month? Are you becoming familiar with them?

Do your moontime patterns flow with changes in energy? Awareness? Needs?

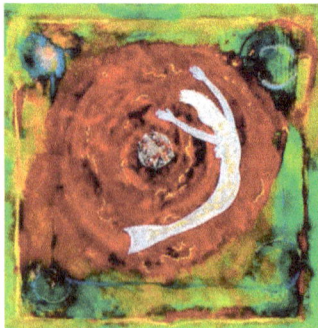

Sun	Mon	Tue	Wed	Thu	Fri	Sat

IDEAS and SUGGESTIONS
to FOLLOW

1. Journal - uncensored thoughts, feelings, reactions to this month's moontime.

_____

_____

_____

_____

_____

2. Dreams and Visions - messages from the unconscious, from your Goddess self.

_____

_____

_____

_____

_____

3. Special self-nurturing reminders - things to do for yourself during your moontime, or during the month, to sustain healing.

_____

_____

_____

_____

_____

4. Preparations needed to create a harmonious moontime - i.e., reminders for child care, appointments to make or cancel, items to purchase, candles to have for a bath.

_____

_____

_____

_____

_____

5. Reminders for food and diet - when to change or eliminate certain foods, take supplements, herbs to have on hand, things to do that release stress.

_____
_____
_____
_____
_____

6. What old beliefs have been uncovered, need to be eliminated or changed?

_____
_____
_____
_____
_____

7. Reminders of activities that will create a harmonious moontime - make an appointment for a massage, walk in nature, get extra sleep, and listen to music that you love.

_____
_____
_____
_____
_____

8. What did your last moontime reveal that will help make the next one more spiritual or bring you closer to your sacred self?

_____
_____
_____
_____
_____

9. Create your own ritual, draw or paint your feelings and/or dreams.

_____
_____
_____
_____
_____

FOCUS #12

THE MOONLODGE or RED TENT

"The fastest way to destroy a tribe is to first destroy the moonlodge"
Native American quote

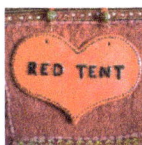

12th month-What is a Moonlodge or Red Tent?

We wembyn lead busy, hectic lives. There's little time left over and if there is, we often feel guilty that we're not doing something important or necessary for someone else.

When does a wombyn get time for herself without feeling guilty or having to be sick? When does a wombyn use time for herself to focus on just herself?

What if each month you decided that you deserved to honor your moontime instead of dreading her? What if you could explain to your partner, boss and children that each month the worker, the partner, the mother needs to be alone to temporarily cut back on some of her responsibilities while she slows down her pace during her moontime? What if businesses had moonlodge rooms like they now have nap rooms? What if they understood that if a wombyn was allowed to honor her cyclic rhythms, she would be replenishing her energy, have less PMS before, less pain during, and would be emerging with more energy, be more productive, happier, and healthier while having more to give? What if everyone realized that if you were given your space to flow in you might even emerge with a vision or realization that could benefit everyone's quality of life?

What if wembyn gave themselves permission to create a moonlodge, red tent, or a place to retreat to for the *soul* purpose of worshipping and honoring their moontimes? What if society as a whole understood this need and honored it? Instead of only *sick days*, what if your place of work also had *red tent or moontime days* and a sanctuary you could retreat to and flow in even for just a short amount of time because everyone knew that when a wombyn has the time to retreat, it creates energy of renewal.

Native American communities, as well as other cultures, do and did honor this sacred wisdom. They created moonlodges for their menstruating wembyn to flow in. Like the red tent, these lodges were separate structures where a menstruating wombyn went during her flow, where she would be safe, cared for and be able to connect with her *self,* needs and sacred inner world.

Moonlodges were huts or teepees where a menstruating wombyn would go to be alone or to be with other wembyn who were menstruating at the same time, a common occurrence amongst indigenous peoples connected to the natural rhythms and phases of the light of the moon. They would bleed onto the earth into soft moss. They would fast, be quiet, dream, pray, receive visions, sing, dance, and be in tune with their flow, allowing it to take them wherever it would. The elders and the fathers would care for the children and relieve the wombyn of their everyday chores. They knew that this was a *holy* time and that their wembyn would return stronger and happier, more empowered and ready to resume life re-energized.

What if modern day wombyn knew that every month she would have the time and space to be alone with herself to drift and dream? What if it was part of her life that once she entered her moontime, she automatically had the opportunity to nourish herself? What if our society supported that because it knew that a wombyn would return stronger and with more to contribute? What if the men or partners in your life supported this for you and realized that your moontime was a reminder to them, too, to go within and see what in their inner worlds needed attention? What if society realized that to offer this support to a moontime wombyn meant a stronger and more sacred society? What if everyone knew and understood that a spiritually empowered wombyn isn't threatening, but has more to give to her family, the work place, her community, and life?

What if we all had the right to visit our moonlodge when we needed to without excuses or justifications? There are many red tents that have been created around the world where a menstruating wombyn can go and flow during her moontime. Check your area and see if there is a red tent available to you. If not, perhaps you can create one.

Here are some ideas that can help create a red tent/moonlodge space.

*Choose a space that will allow you to feel safe, quiet and peaceful. It can be inside or out. It can be your bed piled with red pillows or a cozy couch.

*Prepare ahead to have food, art supplies, things you need to pamper yourself available.

*Allow yourself the time to drift and dream and flow in comfort.

*Recruit others, elders, friends to help with daily needs so you are free to drift and dream.

*Make sure your moonlodge space is comfortable and equipped with the things that make your moontime harmonious.

*Be ready to spend some time separated from your outer life, don't feel guilty about it.

Some moonlodge ideas to think about:

Did you flow in a moonlodge last month?

Will you next month?

Can you create a red tent space for yourself to flow in for at least some part of your moontime, hopefully for the entire time?

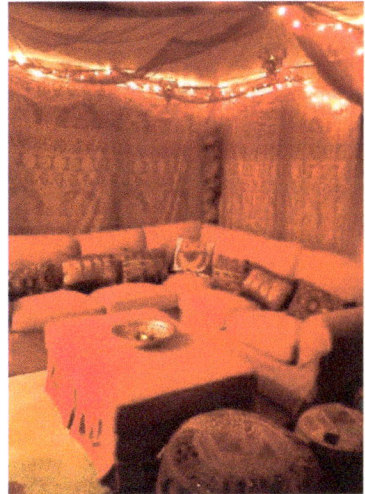

How will you do that? What steps might you need to take to accomplish that goal?

What will your moonlodge be like? What will you equip it with, have ready in it, use it for?

How will you tell your family or the people in your life that you are now flowing in your moonlodge? How will you communicate that you need your separate space and to be quiet?

Use these pages for notes and play.

Use these pages for notes and play.

IDEAS and SUGGESTIONS to FOLLOW

1. Journal - uncensored thoughts, feelings, reactions to this month's moontime.

_____
_____
_____
_____
_____

2. Dreams and Visions - messages from the unconscious, from your Goddess self.

_____
_____
_____
_____
_____

3. Special self-nurturing reminders - things to do for yourself during your moontime, or during the month, to sustain healing.

_____
_____
_____
_____
_____

4. Preparations needed to create a harmonious moontime - i.e., reminders for child care, appointments to make or cancel, items to purchase, candles to have for a bath.

_____
_____
_____
_____
_____

5. Reminders for food and diet - when to change or eliminate certain foods, take supplements, herbs to have on hand, things to do that release stress.

_____

_____

_____

_____

_____

6. What old beliefs have been uncovered, need to be eliminated or changed?

_____

_____

_____

_____

_____

7. Reminders of activities that will create a harmonious moontime - make an appointment for a massage, walk in nature, get extra sleep, and listen to music that you love.

_____

_____

_____

_____

_____

8. What did your last moontime reveal that will help make the next one more spiritual or bring you closer to your sacred self?

_____

_____

_____

_____

_____

9. Create your own ritual, draw or paint your feelings and/or dreams.

_____

_____

_____

_____

_____

FOCUS #13

BECOME an EMPOWERED
MOONTIME WOMBYN

"I will treat wombyn in a sacred manner. The creator gave wombyn the responsibility for bringing new life into the world. Life is sacred, so I will look upon wombyn in a sacred manner."- Native American quote

13ᵗʰ month-Let's Become Moontime Empowered!

As I approached the final part of this workbook, I was magically transported back to the coastal, fishing village where this journey began. It was in a special little town in Mexico that I first opened up to the energy of the lunar reflections of the Goddess and where I began to write this book. Returning to the beginning, to write the ending, was an affirmation to me of the strength and magic that flows within when we dwell in the space of *moontime harmony*.

Moontime is like a flower. She needs care, nurturing, nourishment, and protection in order to thrive and unfold into her full glory and beauty. One's moontime is a path that leads into the flow of the sacred energy of the Divine Feminine or Goddess.

While you flow, you travel along the path of the phases of the moon. You wax and wane through your darkness and light. When you enter into this rhythm, you dance with the Divine. You connect with the Goddess within. Her energy illuminates your darkness, she lights up your shadows. She reveals what is buried. Through this dance of illumination you can cleanse, transform, renew, and let go of the old to flow into the new. Like a snake shedding its old skin to make room for the new one, this Goddess energy of your moontime offers you the monthly opportunity to shed your old to make room for something new.

Moontime is a wombyn's time to care and nurture herself. This often means that there is a need to withdraw from your daily life for a time to be alone. That way you can turn your focus from the outer world to be able to concentrate and listen to your inner world. You remove distractions from the outside, so that the inner can have a safe space in which to surface. It's by resting, dreaming, and retreating that you create harmony and stillness within. When you quiet the tempests of your outer life you can hear what your gentle, soft, quieter, inner voice is whispering. You can cherish this opportunity each month as you cleanse and heal because you are going home to your *self!*

We live in a male-oriented, technological, fast-paced rhythm of life that doesn't know how to slow down or that slowing down is beneficial. There is little room for this feminine flow. The cyclic flow of empty and full, dark and light is not understood or appreciated. Yet, the harmony and healing of one's inner life is necessary in order for there to be harmony and healing of one's outer life. When you understand that attuning to lunar rhythms is the key to flowing in harmony with your moontime rhythm, then you will be able to connect with the sacred Divine Feminine within as well.

Wombyn has this monthly opportunity to remind her. This is a power not a weakness that deserves to be respected, honored and given space, so it can exist as it was created to exist.

A wombyn isn't sick when she is menstruating and shouldn't be made to take sick days if she needs to be alone to care for herself during her flow. **Moontime is not a sickness**.

You can't take more than you put in. People who live close to the earth and garden understand this cycle of sustainable energy. This rhythm of sustainability is also part of the cycle of moontime energy. You need to rest to re-energize. There is a time for outer growth and a time for inner rest. Most of our time we feed our outer life, but then we need to retreat to replenish. When we ignore these rhythms and constantly give, it wears us out. When we ignore these rhythms and constantly take, we wear out Mother Earth. We are wearing out ourselves and Mother Earth. We've forgotten how to balance giving and receiving. It is vitally important that we, as a species, remember this balance and return to this Feminine rhythm because the survival of our earth, children, natural resources, future, and human race depends on living in harmony with this rhythm. Putting the brakes on, at times, does not mean losing profit or power; but can mean insuring the ability to replenish and sustain so we have more and enough for our future.

It's time for wembyn to become fully alive, creative beings, in control of their bodies, sexuality, life choices, and health. It's time to reclaim the wisdom that has been lost or denied, buried or forgotten. Wombyn energetically nourishes life. Globally, we need to return to our

Feminine essence so that we can teach our children and men how to return not only to their feminine lunar nature, but earth-centered balance as well. How else can we live in sacred relationship with Mother Earth who gives us life? How else will we learn how to treat each other with the respect and dignity we all deserve?

Reconnecting with a harmonious moontime is not just about eliminating pain or PMS symptoms, but is also about creating an avenue for the voice of the Divine Feminine to come through as we co-create life on Mother Earth. It is about bringing the Sacred and Divine back into everyday life to rebalance and eliminate the destructive forces that are destroying life itself. Let's not wait any longer to protect Mother Earth so that her life giving energy can thrive and survive. This awareness is now becoming clear to everyone now and a harmonious moontime is a good place for wembyn to start to rediscover this clarity and source of Divinity.

Wombyn is the heart. We yearn to live through our hearts, to love and nurture. Our shared moontime connects us to each other in a soul sisterhood. Wembyn are the ones to ground the Schumann Resonance, or heartbeat of our Earth Mother Gaia, so that life will survive. Our *heavenly waters* of holy, healing blood reminds us each month of that connection.

We know it is time that wombyn and man remember how to exist in balance, beauty and harmony together with each other and with Mother Earth. Gaia's survival depends on this. Life as we know it depends on this. Clean water, oceans, and air depends on this. Living in peace and unity depends on this. The rhythms that create and sustain life depend on this. We can't allow life to be destroyed by ignorance or greedy profiteers who don't understand or care about the essence of the rhythms of life and have no regard or interest in preserving life on this planet. We can't allow our Goddess given gifts and rhythms to be destroyed. We all need to reconnect in harmony.

So I urge every wombyn to find a love for their moontime and to flow with balance and harmony not just for your personal comfort, but for the harmonious balance of life on this planet. May each wombyn unfold her life so she can be in connection with the Divine Feminine, a reflection of Sister Moon. May the wisdom of the lunar moontime light illuminate the way for all beings to live in harmony!

Some things to think about:

What did your moontime illuminate for you last month? What, if anything, returned this month?

What do you need to change to create more harmony in your life? Was this shown to you during your moontime?

How did you nourish yourself this or last moontime?

What special thing did you do for your body, mind or spirit during your last moontime?

Can you affirm the changes that you need for your healing?

Can you affirm that you have special talents and beauty which can be used for a more balanced life?

Has your Divine Feminine voice spoken to you? What did she say?

Can you affirm that your moontime is a harmonious expression of the power and gift of being a Divinely Feminine wombyn? Don't wait, now is the time!

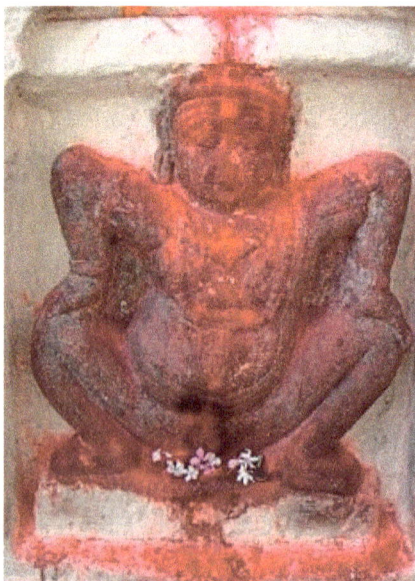

	Sun	Mon	Tue	Wed	Thu	Fri	Sat

IDEAS and SUGGESTIONS to FOLLOW

1. Journal - uncensored thoughts, feelings, reactions to this month's moontime.

_____

_____

_____

_____

_____

2. Dreams and Visions - messages from the unconscious, from your Goddess self.

_____

_____

_____

_____

_____

3. Special self-nurturing reminders - things to do for yourself during your moontime, or during the month, to sustain healing.

_____

_____

_____

_____

_____

4. Preparations needed to create a harmonious moontime - i.e., reminders for child care, appointments to make or cancel, items to purchase, candles to have for a bath.

_____

_____

_____

_____

_____

5. Reminders for food and diet - when to change or eliminate certain foods, take supplements, herbs to have on hand, things to do that release stress.

_____
_____
_____
_____
_____

6. What old beliefs have been uncovered, need to be eliminated or changed?

_____
_____
_____
_____
_____

7. Reminders of activities that will create a harmonious moontime - make an appointment for a massage, walk in nature, get extra sleep, and listen to music that you love.

_____
_____
_____
_____
_____

8. What did your last moontime reveal that will help make the next one more spiritual or bring you closer to your sacred self?

_____
_____
_____
_____

9. Create your own ritual, draw or paint your feelings and/or dreams.

_____
_____
_____
_____
_____

AFTERWORD

I am no longer menstruating and have been in the next phase of my moontime for several years. The rhythms are different, the monthly connection changed, the physical expression gone; but the moontime rhythms still exist and the phases of the moon are still my constant companion and reminder. I still like to chart and follow my inner world's changes, my tides of emotions. The phases of the moon are still my signposts.

Do I still get the physical transformations? No, not in the same ways, but when I pay attention to the lunar phases I do notice both inner and outer rhythms are connected. It is important to me to keep this awareness alive, to follow my cyclic, lunar phases, to stay in touch. When I'm in tune with the moon, I am in tune with me. With the cessation of my moontime flow I have become more vigilant in keeping my lunar awareness alive. I am grateful to be a vessel of this sacred energy.

It is a blessing to know that the energy of the lunar connection can still be a vehicle to remind me to go within to access answers, to visit the garden of the Divine and find avenues of creativity. This is the gift of the Goddess to every wombyn.

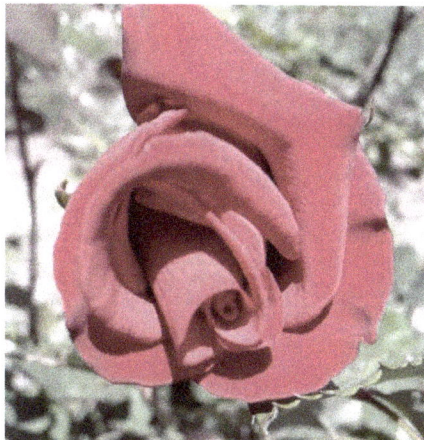

REFERENCES and RESOURCES
RECOMMENDED READINGs-CDs-DVDs
FACEBOOK PAGEs-WEBSITEs

BOOKS

Berger, Gilda, PMS-Premenstrual Syndrome-An Information Book for Teenagers, Women and *Their Friends and Family*, (Alameda, Hunter House Inc., 1991)

Buckley, Thomas C.T. and Alma Gottlieb, *Blood Magic: The Anthropology of Menstruation,* (Berkeley, University of California Press, 1988)

Cameron, Anne, *Daughters of Copper Woman, (*Madeira Park, B.C., Harbor Publishing, LTD (2002)

Diamant, Anita, The Red Tent, (New York, St. Martin's Press, 1997)

Delaney, Lupton, Mary Jane Lupton and Emily Toth, The Curse: A Cultural History of Menstruation, (Illinois, First University of Illinois Press, 1988)

Owen, Lara, Her Blood is Gold: Celebrating the Power of Menstruation, (New York, HarperCollins, 1993)

Eisler, Riane, The Chalice and the Blade, (New York, HarperCollins Publishers, Inc., 1995

Francia, Luisa, Dragon Time: Magic and Mystery of Menstruation, (Woodstock, Ash Tree Publishing, 1991)

George, Demetra, Mysteries of the Dark Moon: The Healing Power of the Dark Goddess, (New York, HarperCollins Publishers, 1992)

Golub, Sharon, Lifting the Curse of Menstruation: A Feminist Appraisal of the Influence of Menstruation on Women's Lives, (Routledge, 1983)

Grahn, Judy, Blood, Bread and Roses: How Menstruation Created the World, (Beacon Press, 1993)

Gray, Miranda, Red Moon, (Fast Print Publishing, 2009)

Hannelore, Barbara, The Moon and You

Pope, Alexandra, The Wild Genie: The Healing Power of Menstruation, (UK, Authors OnLine Ltd, 2013)

Sims, Nao and Nickiah Seeds, Moon Mysteries, (Red Moon Publications, 2011)

Sjoo, Monica and Barbara Mor, The Cosmic Mother: Rediscovering the Religion of the Earth, New York, HarperCollins, 1991

Spider, Songs of Bleeding, (Black Thistle Pr, 1992)

Shuttle, Penelope and Peter Redgrove, The Wise Wound: Myths, Realities, and Meanings of Menstruation, (1988)

Starck, Marcia and Gynne Stem, Women's Medicine Ways:-Cross Cultural Rites of Passage, (The Cross Over Press, 1993)

Starhawk, Spiral Dance, (New York, HarperCollins Publishers, 1999)

Taylor, Dena, The Red Flower-Rethinking Menstruation, (The Blackburn Press, 2003)

Tiwari, Bri. Maya, The Path of Practice: A Woman's Book of Ayurvedic Healing, (Penquin, 2002)

Walker, Barbara G., The Women's Encyclopedia of Myths and Secrets, (New York, HarperCollins, 1996)

Wombwell, Felicity, Goddess Changes: A Personal Guide to Working With the Goddess, (HarperCollins, 1992)

MENARCHE

Dillon, Mary, Flowering Woman: Moontime for Kory, (Sunlight Publishers, 1988)

Hertogs, Rachael, Menarche: A Journey of Womanhood (2013)

Kolkmeyer, Alexandra, The Clear Red Stone: A Myth and the Meaning of Menstruation, (Insight Press, 1982)

Krueger, Katherine, Journey of Young Women, Occupy Menstruation fb page

Torres-Gomez and Erin-Claire Barrow, Cycling to Grandma's House, (Lulu's Publishing Services, 2014)

http://bit.ly/1xokViX, Rojo Menstrual-Muja Cilia, Sophia Style

YOUTUBE, INTERNET

Mary O'Connell radio doc "Seeing Red: A Cultural History of Menstruation"

http://www.cbc.ca/ideas/episodes/2010/06/14/seeing-red-part-1-2-listen/

http://chrysaliswoman.com/1.html/her- moontime-experience-chrysalis-woman.com

www.dailyom.com/articles/2005/375.html

falanstorm.com/she-cycles/empowered sustanence.com/balance-hormones-moon-withgod-dessofsacredsex.com/2013/03/17/the-sacered-power-of-menstrual-blood/

CDs, DVDs, FILM, TALK RADIO, BLOGS, ARTICLES

Brook Medicine Eagle- Moonlodge, CD

Bloodtime, Moontime, Dreamtime-A Poetic Documentary Trilogy by Roberta Cantow, www.originaldigital.net

Bread, Blood and Roses: How Menstruation Created the World- film by Judy Grahn

The Red Tent Movie-www.redtentmovie.com

Woman's Moontime-A Call to Power- Shaman's Drum, spring 1986

She Loves Magazine-www.shelovesmagazine.com

http://adudesguide.com/2014/03/12/lets-talk-menstruation

http://www.blogtalkradio.com/michellemcinnis/2101/09/17/her- blood-is-gold-a-new-way-to-experience-your-monthly-flow

Anea Bogue REALgirl, True Moon http://www.huffingtonpost.ca/anea-bogue/women-menstruation_b_3957384.html

Marguertie Rigoglioso http://divine-feminine.com/the-importance-of-our-menstrual-blood/

Sharon Mc Erlane- "A Call to Power: The Grandmothers Speak", www.periodwise.com

https://awakeningthegoddesswithin.net/13- moon/

Susun Weed, Blood Mysteries, www.herbhealing.com/moonlodge.htm#moon3

http://redtentdirectory.com/create-a-red-tent

http://redtenttemplemovement.com

http://www.youtube.com/watch?v=5EH1d-2aQVg&sns=fb, Sinu Joseph Ted Talk Unwrapping the Gifts of Menstruation

http://www.thefountainoflife.org/sacred-menstruation-reclaiming-our-wise-blood/- The Sacred Power of Menstruation Blood-Seren Swannesha

http:www.shemiranibrahim.com/menstruation-the-sacred- cycle/#sthash.uwonsxqQ.dpuf, Menstruation-The Sacred Cycle-Gina Cloud

The Secret Power of Your Period Revealed- Katherine Smith

Documentary- The Curse

www.karamariaanada.com/blog/2014/8/28/prepare-for-your-period?

www.falanstorm.com/she-cycles/?

http://redtenttempletn.blogspot.com/

The Sacredness of Menstruation in Traditional Tribal Cultures-Sacred Hoop Magazine, winter 2000-2001 edition, Nicholas Noble Wolf

http://naturalshaman.blogspot.com/2012/06/magic-of-menstrual-cycle.html

Sandeep, Bilna- Five Basic Things to Tell Your Son About Periods

WEBSITES

www.susunweed.com

www.womensquest.org

www.womenswaymooncycles.com

www.moonmysteries.com

www.MoontimeRising.com

www.joyouswoman.com

www.Menstrupedia.com

www.deannalam.com

www.ourredtent.com

www.awakeningwomen.com - Awakening Women Institute

www.wisewomanuniversity.org

www.sacred-circle-wisdom.com/grandmother-moon.html

www.grandmotherscouncil.org/

www.daysforgirls.org

http:/www.menstruality.net/

www.mum.org

www.womboflight.com- Bethany Webster

www.IHEARTMYMOONcycle.com

www.globalredtent.com

http://www.menstruation.com.au/

www.redwisom.co.uk

http://theredweb.org - The Red Web Foundation

www.consciousdivas.com

www.redtent.com

www.periodpositive.tumblr.com- Period Positive-Society for Menstrual Cycle Research

FACEBOOK PAGES

Occupy Menstruation

Bloodtime, Moontime, Dreamtime

13 Moons Blood Mysteries, moontime.co.uk

La Tienda Roja, San Diego, Ca.

Guatamala Menstruante

Lunafemina

Moon Mysteries

Women's Way Moon Cycles

The Moon Woman

Mystical Femininity

Women's Quest

Gypsy Muse

Goddess Gathering for Women's Empowerment Forum

Menstruum

Divine Flow

Womb Wisdom

Menstrupedia

About the Author

I was born and raised in Queens and Long Island, N.Y., attended American University and New York University, lived between the suburbs and a modern city until I spent a year traveling in South America two years after I graduated from college.

It was there that I discovered the natural world of the indigenous and that changed my life and the course of its direction.

I fell in love with their crafts, especially pottery and weaving. After my trip was over, I decided to become a potter. I moved and studied pottery at the University of Vermont in Burlington, VT., deepening my love and connection to the earth using pottery as my vehicle. Living in the Green Mountain State brought me closer to nature, where I expanded my love of the natural world.

That connection continued to inspire me. I moved to Quebec, Canada, married, bore 2 children and resided in a small, ski resort village in the country on 37 acres.

Gardening, potting, growing organic food, and raising my 2 children occupied my life until one winter we went traveling to Mexico. Home schooling along the way, we also explored and discovered the fascinating world that Mexico had to offer. It was filled with art, culture, history, markets, and culinary delights.

Our last stop was at a sweet, coastal, jungle, fishing village on the Pacific Coast. I discovered this village before they had phones, internet or electricity. There weren't any paved roads or cars. Walking, riding a mule or a horse was the only form of transportation. The local Mexican and an *expat* community co-existed side by side. Although this unique village now has electricity, phones and internet; it still exists without any paved roads or cars.

I experienced a freedom that living in this natural environment offered to my children, so the following year we moved down for the winter. My children, who were eight and twelve at the time, went to the local schools, learned Spanish and experienced the Mexican culture from their Mexican friends. We were all immersed in the rhythms of this culturally rich and natural world; it was our television screen, entertainment and education.

The ocean tides, lunar light cycles, and seasonal sun all replaced our North American electrical conveniences. There were new plants, new sounds, different animals and insects to learn about, new rhythms to harmonize with that resonated a new awareness inside of us. Here we were immersed in real life, the essence of which I had never experienced before. It was in that environment that I began to flow with my flow.

I fell in love with this lifestyle and lived in this village for eighteen winters. It was there that the Divine Feminine spoke to me. It was during my moontimes that the inspiration and information for this book flowed into my awareness some twenty three years ago.

I wrote the text for this workbook over several moontime cycles, both in this village and in the summers when I returned to my home in Canada. I kept the moontime connection alive. It was in Quebec that I discovered the tapes of Brooke Medicine Eagle. She spoke of the Native American *moontime* and the tradition of using a *moonlodge* to flow in. This was the same experience and information I was discovering when I bled in Mexico, so I immediately incorporated her teachings into my rhythms. This affirmation inspired me to continue on my moontime path and to continue writing this workbook.

Each time I returned to the village in Mexico, another phase of lunar light was illuminated. Finally I felt I'd received all the knowledge I needed in order to flow with and within the Divine *Blood Mysteries*, so I decided to publish my findings.

But the timing wasn't right in 1992, and all my attempts to publish and spread this knowledge went nowhere. So I put my book away until two years ago when the impulse to publish it stirred inside of me again.

I began to look into self-publishing. A friend who recently self-published suggested I check out her publisher. Self-publishing was easy, so why not publish now?

I discovered that the book and movie *The Red Tent* had paved the way to increase menstrual moontime awareness. Red Tents were springing up all over the world. When I discovered the Facebook page Occupy Menstruation, I knew it was time.

As I write this, I am again in that Mexican fishing village, again attuning my spiritual self to the dark and light of the moon. I am thankful to have reconnected with the harmony of my inner rhythms with those of the outer, natural ones. Here, these natural rhythms are unobstructed by electricity, cars or man-made obstacles. Here, I reclaim my thoughts so I can blend and flow with the world of nature, earth, air, and the water that surrounds me. It is in this space and place that I remember my inner Goddess and the truths of the Sacred Divine Feminine.

The connection to the moon is the heart and soul of the moontime, the gift of the Divine that dwells within. You only need to attune to the lunar cycles, listen, and flow with them to find the path that maintains balance and harmony. This gift is always there. Breathe, smile and honor Sister Moon and she will guide you on your journey back home.

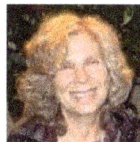

Donna Wolper B.S., C.D., Yelapa, MX, Jan. '15
www.moontimeharmony.com
www.dailyom.com, Healing Your Menstrual Moontime

ABOUT the ARTIST for the BOOK COVER

The cover artist is a self-made, freelance painter and art teacher residing in Santa Cruz, California. She teaches children about art and animals as a job and a hobby. Any spare time she has is devoted to painting and drawing her dreams and the dreams of others. She plans to publish her own comic book and strives to always create beautifully, joyfully and lovingly. Her official assistant and secretary is Poe, her black cat.

Gina Giommi
Santa Cruz, CA
December, 2014

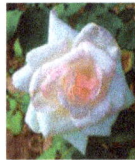

ABOUT the ARTIST for the CALENDAR

I was born and raised in foggy San Francisco and have been looking for sun ever since.

I have lived in Key West, Belize and Guatamala. I now live outside a small Mexican village where I am constantly inspired by natural forms; plant, animal, and human. I particularly believe in human/animal interactions and keeping in touch with the animal spirits within us and without us.

Cata
Yelapa, Jalisco, Mexico
February, 2014

THANK YOUS

I'd like to thank many people who helped me get where I am, not only with helping me with my book, but in my life.

Thank you to my parents whose support allowed me to live in the village in Mexico for many winters, where my muse first spoke to me. Thank you to my muse, where the Goddess whispered her wisdom to me. The unseen powers that have guided me in this magical journey.

Thank you Hadia Benes for doing the beautiful calligraphy on the calendar, reading and editing the text, Jenny D'Angelo for recommending the publisher, giving me tips on publishing, proof reading and editing this manuscript, my first attempt at writing a book. Faye Augustine for her helpful tips, ideas and wonderful art in Focus #12. Claudia Brown for her beautiful Goddess image in Focus #2.

My friends Mae Gene Zimmer and Majalehn La Boheme, constant sources of support for much of my life; my cousin Gary who outfitted my material world with beautiful furniture, an IPad, travel options and more book related ideas to explore; and my brother Richie, whose financial generosity helped make this dream a reality.

Morgan English and Harvey Dosik who gave me stability when my life was shaky, Lynn Gallagher who gave me solace, a bowl of soup and her comfort when I was headed into the unknown.

A special thanks to Susun Weed for taking the time to find and phone me to give me lots of heads ups about book changes that were most necessarily needed to be made! I am ever so grateful.

Angel helpers along the way; Lithia Brigan who opened her red tent and help to me, Amy Jewel who offered to proofread.

And to Super Nifty Gina, the amazing angel and artist, whose artistry and talent pulled this book together!

Zeric Cress the amazing computer wizard who patiently put all this in the proper format with a joyful lightness.

And Alicia Robertson at Robertson Publishing for being so informative and patient.

www.ingramcontent.com/pod-product-compliance
Lightning Source LLC
Chambersburg PA
CBHW061222270326
41927CB00021B/3442